PCOS MEALS SHE NEEDS.

A Cookbook with Recipes That Promote Weight Management, Blood Sugar Control, And Hormonal Balance.

AISHA D. BASSI

Disclaimer

I emphasize consulting with a doctor or registered dietician for personalized guidance throughout pregnancy.

Table of Contents

INTRODUCTION

Welcome to a Delicious Adventure with PCOS!

Congratulations on your pregnancy! This is a magical time filled with excitement and anticipation. But for some women with PCOS, it can also come with a few extra worries.

If you're one of them, take a deep breath and relax – you've got this! This cookbook is designed to be your partner in crime, helping you navigate pregnancy with delicious, PCOS-friendly meals that make you feel fantastic.

Think of this book as your personal chef, whipping up tasty dishes that not only satisfy your cravings but also support your health and the health of your growing baby. Here's why you'll love this adventure:

- **Food as Your Superpower:** We'll show you how to use everyday ingredients to create meals that manage your PCOS symptoms and fuel your body with the nutrients it craves during pregnancy.

- **Bye-Bye Bloat, Hello Energy:** Say goodbye to feeling sluggish and hello to a burst of energy with recipes that promote healthy blood sugar levels and reduce inflammation – naturally!

- **Flavor Without Limits:** Forget bland, boring meals! We've got a treasure trove of delicious recipes that are anything but. From breakfast to dinner and sweet treats, you'll find something to tantalize your taste buds.

- **Easy Does It:** We know you're busy! We've got quick and convenient recipes perfect for fitting healthy meals into your packed schedule.

- **Feel the Difference:** From managing weight gain to regulating periods, witness the power of delicious, PCOS-conscious cooking.

This book is more than just recipes – it's your guide to a happy, healthy pregnancy with PCOS. We'll answer your questions, provide helpful tips, and offer support every step of the way. So, grab your apron, get ready to explore a world of flavor, and let's conquer PCOS together, one delicious meal at a time!

Why This Book is Your Best Friend in the Kitchen:

Planning healthy meals during pregnancy can feel overwhelming, especially with PCOS in the mix. But fear not, mama! This book is here to be your best friend in the kitchen, offering a helping hand (or whisk) throughout your pregnancy journey. Here's how:

- **No More Mystery Meals:** We take the guesswork out of healthy eating with clear, easy-to-follow recipes. No fancy ingredients or complicated techniques – just delicious food that's good for you and your baby.

- **Taming the Cravings:** Pregnancy cravings can be wild! This book is filled with creative recipes that satisfy those cravings while staying true to your PCOS needs. Think satisfying breakfasts that keep you full, lunchtime options that won't leave you sluggish, and delightful dinners that nourish both you and your little one.

- **Your PCOS Whisperer:** We understand the unique challenges PCOS can bring to pregnancy. This book offers recipes and tips specifically tailored to manage PCOS symptoms, like blood sugar control and inflammation. It's like having a PCOS whisperer in the kitchen, guiding you towards healthy choices.

- **Time-Saving Superhero:** We get it – you're growing a tiny human! Time is precious. This book is packed with quick and convenient recipes that can be whipped up in no time, even on the busiest days. Plus, many recipes offer leftover magic, perfect for those days you just don't feel like cooking.

- **The Flavor Fairy:** Let's face it, bland food is no fun! This book is your ticket to flavortown. We've got a vibrant collection of recipes bursting with taste, ensuring you enjoy every bite while staying on track with your PCOS goals.

Think of this book as your personal cheerleader in the kitchen, encouraging you to make healthy choices that are both delicious and supportive of your PCOS and pregnancy. So, ditch the stress and frustration – let's cook up some magic together!

CHAPTER 1: What is PCOS and How Does it Affect You?

Understanding Your Superpower:

Congratulations on your pregnancy! This is a time of incredible change and wonder. But for some mamas with PCOS, it can also come with a few extra questions. This chapter is here to be your friendly guide, explaining PCOS in a clear and simple way, so you can focus on the joy of your pregnancy journey.

What is PCOS?

PCOS, or polycystic ovary syndrome, is a hormonal imbalance that affects many women. It happens when your ovaries produce more androgen than usual (androgen is a male hormone that women also have in small amounts). This can cause a few different symptoms, but the most common ones include:

- **Irregular Periods:** You might have periods that come and go unpredictably, or you might skip them altogether.

- **Unwanted Guests:** Excess androgen can lead to unwanted hair growth on your face and body.

- **Acne Attack:** Androgen can also contribute to pesky breakouts.

- **Trouble Getting Pregnant:** PCOS can sometimes make it harder to conceive.

How Does PCOS Affect Pregnancy?

The good news is that plenty of women with PCOS have healthy pregnancies! However, PCOS can sometimes affect pregnancy in a few ways:

- **Blood Sugar Blues:** PCOS can make it harder for your body to use insulin, a hormone that helps regulate blood sugar. This is called insulin resistance, and it can increase your risk of gestational diabetes during pregnancy.

- **Weight Gain Worries:** PCOS can sometimes make it harder to lose weight or keep it off. This can be a concern during pregnancy, as healthy weight management is important for both you and your baby.

Don't Panic!

This chapter might have thrown a few new terms your way, but remember, knowledge is power! Understanding PCOS can help you manage it and have a healthy pregnancy. The rest of this book will be your partner in crime, providing delicious recipes and tips to navigate PCOS while you nourish yourself and your growing baby.

We've Got Your Back!

If you have any questions or concerns about PCOS and pregnancy, talk to your doctor. They are there to support you and help you have a happy, healthy journey. Now, let's get cooking and create some delicious memories (and meals) together!

CHAPTER 2: Food as Medicine: How Diet Can Improve PCOS Symptoms

Fueling Your Superpower:

Pregnancy is a time of incredible transformation, and your body needs the right fuel to thrive. This chapter deep into the amazing world of food as medicine, showing you how simple dietary changes can make a big difference in managing your PCOS symptoms and supporting a healthy pregnancy.

Food Fights Back!

Think of food as your personal superhero sidekick! The choices you make at mealtimes can actually help fight back against some of the common symptoms of PCOS, like:

- **Blood Sugar Blues:** Remember how we talked about insulin resistance in Chapter 1? Well, certain foods can help your body use insulin more effectively, keeping your blood sugar levels in check. This is especially important during pregnancy to reduce the risk of gestational diabetes.

- **Inflammation Frustration:** Chronic inflammation can be a sneaky culprit behind some PCOS symptoms. But worry not! Certain foods have powerful anti-inflammatory properties, helping to reduce inflammation and promote overall well-being.

- **Weight Management Woes:** Managing weight gain is crucial for a healthy pregnancy, and PCOS can sometimes make it tricky. But fear not, mama! This chapter will introduce you to delicious, filling foods that can help you maintain a healthy weight without feeling deprived.

The PCOS Power Plate:

Imagine a plate bursting with colorful, delicious ingredients – that's your PCOS Power Plate! This chapter will introduce you to the key food groups that form the foundation of a PCOS-friendly diet, perfect for pregnancy:

- **Veggie Superstars:** Vibrant vegetables are packed with essential vitamins, minerals, and fiber – all superstars for your health. We'll show you creative ways to incorporate more veggies into your meals, making them both delicious and satisfying.

- **Lean Protein Powerhouses:** Protein is essential for building and repairing tissues, which is super important during pregnancy! Lean protein sources like chicken, fish, beans, and lentils will keep you feeling full and energized.

- **Healthy Fat Fantastic:** Don't be afraid of healthy fats! They play a vital role in hormone balance, cell growth, and keeping you feeling satisfied. We'll show you delicious sources of healthy fats like avocado, nuts, seeds, and olive oil.

- **Whole Grain Wonders:** Whole grains are a fantastic source of complex carbohydrates, which provide sustained energy throughout the day. They'll also keep you feeling fuller for longer, helping to manage cravings.

The Recipe for Success:

This chapter isn't just about what to eat – it's about how to make healthy eating work for you during pregnancy. We'll provide tips on:

- **Planning Power:** Planning your meals ahead of time can be a lifesaver, especially when you're feeling tired or busy. We'll offer simple meal planning strategies to keep you on track.

- **Snacking Savvy:** Pregnancy cravings can be real! We'll show you how to choose healthy snacks that satisfy your cravings without derailing your PCOS goals.

- **Portion Perfection:** Knowing how much to eat is important for both you and your baby. We'll provide guidance on portion control to ensure you're getting the nutrients you both needs.

By embracing food as medicine and incorporating the tips in this chapter, you can feel empowered to manage your PCOS symptoms and nourish your body for a happy, healthy pregnancy. Now, let's get cooking and create some delicious meals that fuel your amazing journey!

CHAPTER 3: Building a Balanced Plate for PCOS Management

The PCOS Power Plate in Action:

Now that you've met the superstar ingredients of the PCOS Power Plate in Chapter 2, it's time to put them into action! This chapter dives into the nitty-gritty of building balanced meals that manage your PCOS symptoms and support a thriving pregnancy.

Balancing Act:

Think of your plate as a colorful masterpiece! Each section plays a crucial role in creating a balanced and delicious meal that benefits both you and your baby. Here's how to fill it up:

- **Half Your Plate for Veggies:** Vegetables are champions of the PCOS Power Plate! They're packed with essential vitamins, minerals, and fiber that keep your body functioning at its best. Aim to fill half your plate with a vibrant rainbow of veggies – think leafy greens, broccoli, peppers, sweet potatoes, and whatever else tickles your taste buds. We'll show you creative ways to incorporate them into every meal, from roasted veggies to breakfast scrambles and veggie-packed pasta dishes.

- **A Quarter Lean Protein Powerhouse:** Protein is the building block of life, and it's especially important during pregnancy! Aim for a quarter of your plate to be filled with lean protein sources like chicken, fish, beans, lentils, and tofu. These will keep you feeling full and energized throughout the day.

- **A Quarter Whole Grain Wonders:** Whole grains are another champion on the PCOS Power Plate! They offer a slow and steady release of energy, helping you manage cravings and blood sugar levels. Fill the remaining quarter of your plate with whole grains like brown rice, quinoa, whole-wheat bread, or whole-grain pasta.

- **Healthy Fat Fantastic:** Don't forget the healthy fats! They play a crucial role in hormone balance, cell growth, and keeping you feeling satisfied. Add a sprinkle of healthy fats to your plate with options like avocado slices, a drizzle of olive oil, nuts and seeds sprinkled on your salad, or a dollop of nut butter with your fruit.

The Art of Variety:

Variety is the spice of life, and it's also key to a healthy PCOS-friendly diet! This chapter will provide tons of inspiration with:

- **Mix and Match Magic:** We'll show you how to mix and match the power plate ingredients to create endless possibilities for delicious and nutritious meals.

- **Seasonal Symphony:** Embrace the bounty of each season! We'll offer tips on incorporating seasonal fruits and vegetables into your meals, making them both delicious and affordable.

- **Spice It Up!** Don't be shy with herbs and spices! They add flavor, depth, and a touch of magic to your meals while often boasting additional health benefits. We'll give you suggestions on using herbs and spices to create exciting flavor profiles.

Beyond the Plate:

Building a balanced plate is a great foundation, but this chapter goes beyond just food. We'll also provide tips on:

- **Hydration Hero:** Water is essential for everyone, and even more so during pregnancy. We'll remind you of the importance of staying hydrated and offer tips on making water more exciting.

- **Portion Perfection:** Knowing how much to eat is important for both you and your baby. We'll provide guidance on portion control to ensure you're getting the nutrients you both need without overdoing it.

- **Mindful Eating:** Eating mindfully can be a powerful tool for managing cravings and preventing overeating. We'll offer tips on practicing mindful eating and savoring your food.

By following the tips in this chapter and filling your plate with the power plate superstars, you can create delicious, balanced meals that support your PCOS management and nourish your body for a happy, healthy pregnancy! Now, let's get cooking and explore some delicious recipes that put your PCOS Power Plate into action!

CHAPTER 4: Filling Your Plate with Powerhouse Foods:

Fueling Your Body with the Best:

Now that you've mastered the art of building a balanced plate in Chapter 3, it's time to zoom in on the superstar ingredients themselves! This chapter dives deep into each category of the PCOS Power Plate, giving you the lowdown on the best whole grains, lean proteins, healthy fats, and vibrant fruits and veggies to fuel your amazing journey.

Whole Grains and Complex Carbs: Slow and Steady Wins the Race!

Whole grains are the unsung heroes of the PCOS Power Plate. Unlike refined carbohydrates, which can cause blood sugar spikes, whole grains offer a slow and steady release of energy, keeping you feeling full and satisfied for longer. They're also packed with essential nutrients like fiber, B vitamins, and minerals, all crucial for a healthy pregnancy.

Here are some whole-grain champions to add to your plate:

- **Brown Rice:** A classic choice with a nutty flavor, perfect for bowls, stir-fries, and pilafs.

- **Quinoa:** This protein-rich grain offers a complete amino acid profile, making it a fantastic plant-based protein source. Enjoy it in salads, bowls, or as a side dish.

- **Whole-Wheat Bread:** Choose whole-wheat bread over white bread for your toast or sandwiches. Look for varieties with at least 3 grams of fiber per slice.

- **Whole-Grain Pasta:** Swap out your regular pasta for whole-wheat versions. They cook up just as well and offer a satisfying fiber boost.

- **Oats:** A powerhouse breakfast option, oats are packed with fiber and keep you feeling full for hours. Enjoy them with berries, nuts, and a drizzle of honey.

Lean Protein Powerhouses: Building Blocks for Life!

Protein is the building block of life, and it's especially important during pregnancy as your baby grows and develops. Lean protein sources provide sustained energy, keep you feeling full, and help regulate blood sugar levels.

Here are some lean protein powerhouses to add to your plate:

- **Chicken and Turkey:** These versatile proteins can be baked, grilled, or roasted and enjoyed in a variety of dishes. Choose lean cuts like chicken breasts or turkey tenderloins.

- **Fish:** Salmon, tuna, and other fatty fish are packed with omega-3 fatty acids, which are crucial for brain development and overall health. Aim for 2-3 servings of fish per week.

- **Beans and Lentils:** These plant-based protein sources are budget-friendly and offer a good dose of fiber too. Enjoy them in soups, salads, or as a main course.

- **Tofu and Tempeh:** These vegetarian protein options are perfect for meatless meals. They can be marinated, baked, or crumbled and used in various dishes.

Healthy Fats for Hormone Balance: Don't Be Afraid of Fat!

Healthy fats are essential for hormone balance, cell growth, and keeping you feeling satisfied. They also help your body absorb certain vitamins. Don't be afraid to incorporate healthy fats into your diet!

Here are some healthy fat superstars to add to your plate:

- **Avocado:** This creamy fruit is loaded with healthy monounsaturated fats, fiber, and essential vitamins. Enjoy it sliced on toast, in salads, or mashed into guacamole.

- **Nuts and Seeds:** Almonds, walnuts, chia seeds, and flaxseeds are fantastic sources of healthy fats, fiber, and protein. Sprinkle them on salads, yogurt, or oatmeal, or enjoy them as a healthy snack.

- **Olive Oil:** A staple in Mediterranean cuisine, olive oil is rich in monounsaturated fats and antioxidants. Use it for drizzling, dressing salads, or sauteing vegetables.

- **Fatty Fish:** As mentioned earlier, salmon, tuna, and other fatty fish are packed with omega-3 fatty acids, which are crucial for brain development and overall health.

Vibrant Fruits and Veggies: Nature's Candy!

Fruits and vegetables are bursting with essential vitamins, minerals, fiber, and antioxidants, all crucial for a healthy pregnancy. They come in a rainbow of colors, each with unique health benefits.

Here's how to fill your plate with veggie and fruit power:

- **Aim for Variety:** Think of your plate as a colorful masterpiece! Incorporate a variety of fruits and vegetables throughout the day.

- **Leafy Greens Lead the Way:** Leafy greens like spinach, kale, and swiss chard are packed with nutrients like folate, iron, and calcium – all essential for pregnancy.

- **Rainbow Power:** Each color of the rainbow offers unique health benefits. Aim for a variety of colors on your plate, from red tomatoes and peppers to orange sweet potatoes and carrots, yellow bell peppers and corn, green leafy greens and broccoli, to vibrant purple eggplants and blueberries.

- **Don't Forget the Frozen Section:** Frozen fruits and vegetables are flash-frozen at peak freshness, locking in nutrients. They're a convenient and affordable way to add variety to your meals.

- **Sweet Treats Done Right:** While fruits are naturally sweet, limit sugary fruits like mangoes and grapes. Opt for berries, apples, pears, and citrus fruits for a satisfying sweetness without a blood sugar spike.

By incorporating these powerhouse foods into your diet, you'll be fueling your body with the essential nutrients it needs to manage PCOS and support a healthy pregnancy. The next chapter will look into how to plan, create and keep pantry staples for PCOS Success! So, get ready to explore a world of flavor and embark on a culinary adventure that nourishes both you and your growing baby!

CHAPTER 5: Pantry Staples for PCOS Success

Your PCOS Powerhouse Pantry:

Imagine your pantry as your secret weapon in the fight against PCOS symptoms and supporting a healthy pregnancy! By stocking it with the right essentials, you'll be setting yourself up for success in creating delicious and nutritious meals throughout your pregnancy journey.

The Essential All-Stars:

These pantry staples are your go-to ingredients for whipping up quick, healthy meals that are perfect for busy days:

- **Canned Beans and Lentils:** A budget-friendly protein and fiber powerhouse. Stock up on varieties like kidney beans, chickpeas, black beans, and lentils. They're perfect for adding to salads, soups, or creating vegetarian main courses.

- **Whole-Grain Pastas and Rice:** Choose brown rice, quinoa, whole-wheat pasta, and other whole-grain options for a slow and steady release of energy.

- **Canned Fish:** Tuna, salmon, and sardines are packed with omega-3 fatty acids and protein. They're a convenient option for quick lunches or protein additions to salads.

- **Nut Butters:** Opt for natural peanut butter, almond butter, or cashew butter for a healthy dose of protein, healthy fats, and fiber. Enjoy them on whole-wheat toast, with apple slices, or as a base for homemade salad dressings.

- **Dried Fruits and Nuts:** Keep a variety of nuts and seeds like almonds, walnuts, chia seeds, and flaxseeds on hand for a quick and healthy snack or to add protein and fiber to yogurt, oatmeal, or salads. Choose dried fruits like cranberries, raisins, and cherries for a touch of natural sweetness, but be mindful of portion sizes.

- **Healthy Oils:** Stock up on olive oil, avocado oil, or grapeseed oil for healthy fats and cooking needs.

- **Vinegars and Spices:** A sprinkle of herbs and spices can transform a simple dish. Keep a variety of your favorites on hand, like garlic powder, onion powder, dried herbs like oregano and basil, and different types of pepper. Apple cider vinegar and balsamic vinegar are great for salad dressings and marinades.

- **Canned or Frozen Veggies:** These are lifesavers for busy days and ensure you always have veggie options on hand. Choose options with no added sodium for the healthiest choices.

Beyond the Basics:

This chapter goes beyond the basic staples and introduces you to some additional pantry friends that can add variety and flavor to your PCOS-friendly meals:

- **Whole-Grain Bread and Crackers:** Choose whole-wheat bread or whole-grain crackers for healthy snacking options or bases for sandwiches.

- **Oatmeal:** A fantastic breakfast option, oatmeal keeps you feeling full for hours. Stock up on quick oats or rolled oats, depending on your preference.

- **Healthy Grains:** Explore options like quinoa flakes, barley, or bulgur wheat for added variety in your whole-grain repertoire.

- **Dried Beans and Grains:** While canned options are convenient, consider keeping some dried beans and grains on hand for making larger batches or for meals requiring a more specific texture.

- **Low-Sugar Sweeteners:** If you crave a touch of sweetness, explore options like stevia, monk fruit sweetener, or a small amount of pure maple syrup.

Pantry Power Tips:

This chapter also equips you with helpful tips for keeping your pantry stocked and organized for PCOS success:

- **Plan Your Meals:** Planning your meals ahead of time allows you to create a grocery list and avoid impulse purchases. This ensures you have the ingredients on hand to make healthy PCOS-friendly meals.

- **Read Labels Carefully:** Not all whole-grain products are created equal. Get in the habit of reading food labels and choosing options with high fiber content and minimal added sugars.

- **Buy in Bulk (Smartly):** Buying certain staples like whole-grain pasta, brown rice, or nut butters in bulk can save you money in the long run. However, only buy in bulk for items you'll use before they expire.

- **First In, First Out (FIFO):** Rotate your pantry staples regularly to ensure you're using the older items first and prevent anything from expiring in the back of the shelf.

- **Embrace Variety:** Don't get stuck in a rut! Experiment with different pantry staples to create exciting and flavorful meals throughout your pregnancy.

By stocking your pantry with these PCOS powerhouses and following the tips in this chapter, you'll be well on your way to creating delicious and nutritious meals that support your PCOS management and nourish your body for a happy, healthy pregnancy! Now, get ready to explore a world of flavor as we start to look into delicious recipes in the next chapter!

CHAPTER 6: Breakfast Recipes

Fueling Your Morning:

Breakfast is the most important meal of the day, and that's especially true during pregnancy! This chapter is packed with delicious and satisfying PCOS-friendly breakfast ideas that will keep you energized and feeling your best all morning long.

We've got options for every taste and time crunch, including:

- **Quick and Easy Ideas:** Perfect for busy mornings when you're short on time.

- **Sweet and Savory Choices:** Something to satisfy every craving, whether you're a sweet tooth or a savory seeker.

- **Protein-Packed Powerhouses:** Breakfasts that keep you feeling full and energized throughout the morning.

Each recipe includes:

- A brief description of the dish
- Preparation and cooking duration
- Number of servings
- Ingredient list
- Step-by-step instructions with easy-to-follow guidance
- Nutritional information, including calories, carbohydrates, protein, and fat

Servings: 01

Cooking Time:

10 Minutes

1. Scrumptious Scrambled Eggs with

This protein-packed breakfast is bursting with flavor and keeps you feeling full for hours.

Ingredients	Cooking Instructions
1. 2 large eggs 2. 1 tablespoon unsweetened almond milk 3. 1/2 cup chopped fresh spinach 4. 1/4 cup crumbled feta cheese 5. 1/4 teaspoon dried oregano 6. Salt and pepper to taste 7. Non-stick cooking spray	1. In a small bowl, whisk together the eggs and almond milk. Season with a pinch of salt and pepper. 2. Heat a non-stick skillet over medium heat. Coat the pan with cooking spray. 3. Add the spinach to the pan and cook until wilted, about 1 minute. 4. Pour the egg mixture into the pan with the spinach. Let it cook for a minute, then gently scramble the eggs with a spatula until cooked through to your desired consistency. 5. Remove from heat and crumble the feta cheese over the top. Sprinkle with oregano and serve immediately. • **<u>Nutritional Information (per serving):</u>** Calories: 280, Carbohydrates: 5g, Protein: 18g, Fat: 18g

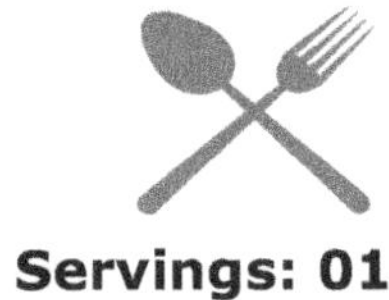

Servings: 01

Cooking Time:

5 Minutes

2. Berriedlicious Overnight Oats

Prep this breakfast the night before for a quick and delicious grab-and-go option in the morning.

Ingredients	Cooking Instructions
1. 1/2 cup rolled oats 2. 1/2 cup unsweetened almond milk (or other milk of your choice) 3. 1/4 cup plain Greek yogurt 4. 1/4 cup mixed berries (fresh or frozen) 5. 1 tablespoon chia seeds 6. 1/2 teaspoon ground cinnamon 7. Pinch of stevia or monk fruit sweetener (optional)	1. In a jar or container, combine the rolled oats, almond milk, Greek yogurt, berries, chia seeds, and cinnamon. Stir well. 2. If using stevia or monk fruit sweetener, add a pinch to taste. 3. Cover the jar securely and refrigerate overnight. 4. In the morning, give it a quick stir and enjoy! **Nutritional Information (per serving):** Calories:300, Carbohydrates: 35g, Protein: 10g, Fat: 10g

Servings: 01

Cooking Time:

5 Minutes prep

3. Sunshine Smoothie

This vibrant smoothie is packed with vitamins, protein, and healthy fats to keep you energized all morning.

Ingredients	Cooking Instructions
1. 1 cup frozen mango chunks 2. ½ cup baby spinach 3. ½ banana 4. ¼ cup plain Greek yogurt 5. ¼ cup unsweetened almond milk 6. 1 tablespoon chia seeds 7. 1 teaspoon fresh lime juice	1. Combine all ingredients in a blender and blend until smooth and creamy. 2. Enjoy immediately! **Nutritional Information (per serving):** Calories: 320, Carbohydrates: 40g, Protein: 12g, Fat: 10g

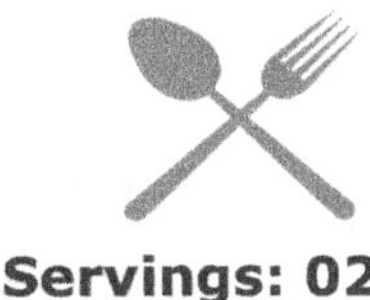

Servings: 02

Cooking Time:

30 Minutes

4. Savory Veggie Frittata

This protein and veggie-packed frittata is a hearty and satisfying breakfast option.

Ingredients	Cooking Instructions
1. ½ tablespoon olive oil 2. ½ cup chopped red bell pepper 3. ½ cup chopped broccoli florets 4. ¼ cup chopped onion 5. 4 large eggs, beaten 6. ½ cup crumbled feta cheese 7. ¼ cup chopped fresh parsley 8. Salt and pepper to taste	1. Preheat oven to 375°F (190°C). Grease a small oven-safe skillet. 2. Heat olive oil in a skillet over medium heat. Add the bell pepper, broccoli, and onion. Sauté for 5 minutes, or until softened. 3. In a large bowl, whisk together the eggs, feta cheese, and parsley. Season with salt and pepper. 4. Pour the egg mixture into the skillet with the vegetables. Stir gently to combine. 5. Bake in the preheated oven for 20-25 minutes, or until the eggs are set and the center is cooked through. 6. Let cool slightly before serving. **Nutritional Information (per serving):** Calories: 300, Carbohydrates: 8g, Protein: 20g, Fat: 18g (without almonds and honey)

Servings: 02

Cooking Time:

20 Minutes

5. Power Up Pancakes

These whole-wheat pancakes are packed with protein and fiber to keep you feeling full and satisfied.

Ingredients	Cooking Instructions
1. 1 cup whole-wheat flour 2. 1 teaspoon baking powder 3. ½ teaspoon ground cinnamon 4. ¼ teaspoon salt 5. 1 cup unsweetened almond milk (or other milk of your choice) 6. 1 large egg 7. 1 tablespoon melted coconut oil	1. In a large bowl, whisk together the flour, baking powder, cinnamon, and salt. 2. In a separate bowl, whisk together the almond milk, egg, and melted coconut oil. 3. Pour the wet ingredients into the dry ingredients and whisk until just combined. Do not overmix. 4. Heat a lightly greased griddle or skillet over medium heat. 5. Pour ¼ cup batter per pancake onto the griddle. Cook for 2-3 minutes per side, or until golden brown and cooked through. 6. Serve immediately with your favorite toppings like fresh berries, chopped nuts, or a drizzle of pure maple syrup.

Nutritional Information (per serving):

Calories: 300, Carbohydrates: 35g, Protein: 12g, Fat: 10g

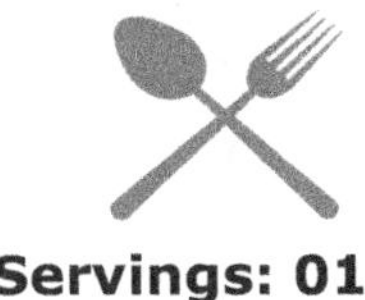

Servings: 01

Cooking Time:

5 Minutes

6. Chia Pudding Perfection

This creamy and satisfying chia pudding is a great meal-prep option for busy mornings.

Ingredients	Cooking Instructions
1. 1/3 cup chia seeds 2. 1 cup unsweetened almond milk (or other milk of your choice) 3. 1/4 cup plain Greek yogurt 4. 1/4 cup chopped fresh berries 5. 1 tablespoon sliced almonds 6. 1/2 teaspoon vanilla extract 7. Pinch of ground cinnamon	1. In a jar or container, combine the chia seeds, almond milk, Greek yogurt, berries, almonds, vanilla extract, and cinnamon. Stir well. 2. Cover the jar securely and refrigerate overnight. 3. In the morning, give it a quick stir and enjoy! **Nutritional Information (per serving):** Calories: 350, Carbohydrates: 30g, Protein: 15g, Fat: 15g

Servings: 02

Cooking Time:

15 Minutes

7. Spicy Black Bean Scramble

This protein-rich scramble is full of flavor and keeps you feeling energized.

Ingredients	Cooking Instructions
1. 1 tablespoon olive oil 2. ½ cup chopped red onion 3. ½ cup chopped green bell pepper 4. 1 clove garlic, minced 5. 1 can (15 oz) black beans, rinsed and drained 6. 2 large eggs, beaten 7. ¼ cup crumbled feta cheese 8. 1 tablespoon chopped fresh cilantro 9. ½ teaspoon chili powder 10. ¼ teaspoon smoked paprika 11. Salt and pepper to taste	1. Heat olive oil in a skillet over medium heat. Add the onion, bell pepper, and garlic. Sauté for 5 minutes, or until softened. 2. Add the black beans to the pan and cook for an additional minute. 3. Push the bean mixture to one side of the pan. Pour the beaten eggs into the empty side of the pan. Scramble the eggs until almost cooked through. 4. Fold the bean mixture into the scrambled eggs. 5. Sprinkle with feta cheese, cilantro, chili powder, and smoked paprika. Season with salt and pepper to taste. 6. Cook for an additional minute or two, or until the cheese is melted and the eggs are cooked through. 7. Serve immediately with avocado slices and whole-wheat toast (optional).

<u>Nutritional Information (per serving):</u>

Calories: 350, Carbohydrates: 30g, Protein: 20g, Fat: 15g

Servings: 01

Cooking Time: 20 Minutes

8. Sweet Potato Power Toast

This recipe takes your average avocado toast up a notch with the addition of vitamin A-rich sweet potato.

Ingredients	Cooking Instructions
1. ½ medium sweet potato, peeled and diced 2. ½ tablespoon olive oil 3. ½ avocado, sliced 4. 1 slice whole-wheat toast 5. 1 large egg 6. 1 tablespoon crumbled feta cheese 7. Pinch of dried oregano 8. Salt and pepper to taste	1. Preheat oven to 400°F (200°C). Toss the diced sweet potato with olive oil and a pinch of salt and pepper. Spread on a baking sheet and roast for 15-20 minutes, or until tender. 2. While the sweet potato roasts, cook your egg however you like it (fried, scrambled, poached). 3. Toast your whole-wheat bread. 4. Spread the avocado slices on the toast. Top with the roasted sweet potato and cooked egg. 5. Crumble feta cheese over the top and sprinkle with oregano. Season with additional salt and pepper to taste.

<u>Nutritional Information (per serving):</u>

Calories: 350, Carbohydrates: 30g, Protein: 15g, Fat: 15g

Servings: 01

**Cooking Time:
15 Minutes**

9. Breakfast Buddha Bowl

This recipe offers a base and endless topping possibility for a protein-packed and visually appealing breakfast.

Ingredients	Cooking Instructions
1. ½ cup cooked quinoa 2. ½ cup chopped baby spinach 3. ¼ cup chopped cucumber 4. ¼ cup cherry tomatoes, halved 5. 2 tablespoons crumbled feta cheese 6. 2 tablespoons chopped walnuts 7. 1 hard-boiled egg, sliced For the dressing: - 1 tablespoon olive oil - 1 tablespoon lemon juice - Pinch of dried oregano - Salt and pepper to taste	1. In a bowl, combine the cooked quinoa, spinach, cucumber, cherry tomatoes, feta cheese, walnuts, and sliced egg. 2. In a separate jar or small bowl, whisk together the olive oil, lemon juice, oregano, salt, and pepper for the dressing. 3. Drizzle the dressing over the breakfast bowl ingredients. 4. Toss to coat and enjoy! **Nutritional Information (per serving):** Calories: 400, Carbohydrates: 40g, Protein:20g, Fat: 15g

Servings: 01　　　　**Cooking Time:
10 Minutes**

10. Greek Yogurt Parfait Perfection

A classic and satisfying breakfast option with endless flavor variations.

Ingredients	Cooking Instructions
<ul><li>½ cup plain Greek yogurt</li><li>¼ cup granola (choose a low-sugar option)</li><li>¼ cup fresh berries</li><li>1 tablespoon chopped nuts (almonds, walnuts, or pecans)</li><li>Drizzle of honey (optional)</li></ul>	1. In a bowl or parfait glass, layer the Greek yogurt, granola, berries, and nuts. 2. Drizzle with honey for an extra touch of sweetness (optional). **<u>Nutritional Information (per serving):</u>** Calories: 300, Carbohydrates: 30g, Protein: 15g, Fat: 10g

Servings: 01

**Cooking Time:
15 Minutes**

11. Hearty Breakfast Burrito

Perfect for busy mornings, this protein-packed burrito keeps you feeling full and satisfied.

Ingredients	Cooking Instructions
• 1 whole-wheat tortilla • 2 scrambled eggs • ¼ cup chopped black beans • 2 tablespoons shredded cheese (cheddar or Monterey Jack) • ¼ cup chopped salsa • 1 tablespoon chopped avocado (optional)	1. Warm a whole-wheat tortilla in a skillet or microwave. 2. Scramble your eggs until cooked through. 3. Spread the scrambled eggs over the warmed tortilla. 4. Top with black beans, cheese, salsa, and avocado (if using). 5. Fold the tortilla into a burrito and enjoy! **<u>Nutritional Information (per serving):</u>** Calories: 350, Carbohydrates: 30g, Protein: 20g, Fat: 15g

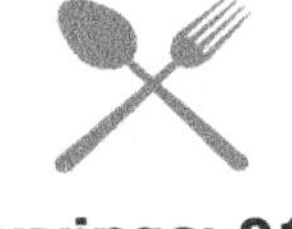

Servings: 01

**Cooking Time:
10 Minutes**

12. Tropical Smoothie Bowl

This vibrant smoothie bowl is packed with antioxidants and keeps you cool on warm mornings.

Ingredients	Cooking Instructions
<ul><li>1 cup frozen mango chunks</li><li>½ cup frozen pineapple chunks</li><li>½ banana</li><li>½ cup unsweetened almond milk (or other milk of your choice)</li><li>¼ cup plain Greek yogurt</li></ul>**Toppings (choose your favorites):** - Granola - Fresh berries - Chopped nuts - Shredded coconut	er the frozen mango, pineapple, banana, almond ːek yogurt in a blender until smooth and creamy. ɔothie into a bowl. orite toppings and enjoy! **Nutritional Information (per serving):** Calories: 350, Carbohydrates: 45g, Protein: 10g, Fat: 10g

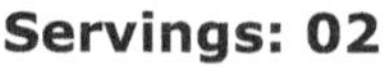

Servings: 02   **Cooking Time: 20 Minutes**

13. Protein Pancakes with Almond Butter Power

These protein-packed pancakes are perfect for satisfying your sweet tooth while keeping you feeling full.

Ingredients	Cooking Instructions
<ul><li>1 cup cottage cheese</li><li>1 large egg</li><li>½ cup rolled oats</li><li>1 teaspoon baking powder</li><li>¼ teaspoon ground cinnamon</li><li>2 tablespoons unsweetened almond butter</li><li>1 tablespoon milk (optional, if batter seems too thick)</li></ul>	1. In a blender or food processor, blend together the cottage cheese, egg, rolled oats, baking powder, and cinnamon until smooth. 2. Stir in the almond butter until just combined. If the batter seems too thick, add a tablespoon of milk to thin it out. 3. Heat a lightly greased griddle or skillet over medium heat. 4. Pour ¼ cup batter per pancake onto the griddle. Cook for 2-3 minutes per side, or until golden brown and cooked through. 5. Serve immediately with your favorite toppings like fresh berries, chopped nuts, or a drizzle of pure maple syrup.

<u>Nutritional Information (per serving):</u>
Calories: 300, Carbohydrates: 30g, Protein: 20g, Fat: 10g

Servings: 01   **Cooking Time:
20 Minutes**

14. Eggs Benedict with a Twist

This recipe uses whole-wheat English muffins and Canadian bacon for a more PCOS-friendly twist on a classic dish.

Ingredients	Cooking Instructions
<ul><li>1 whole-wheat English muffin, toasted</li><li>2 slices Canadian bacon</li><li>2 large eggs</li></ul>**For the hollandaise sauce (light version):**<ul><li>1 egg yolk</li><li>1 tablespoon lemon juice</li><li>1/4 cup low-fat Greek yogurt</li><li>Pinch of cayenne pepper</li><li>Salt and pepper to taste</li></ul>	1. Poach the eggs according to your preferred method. 2. While the eggs are poaching, prepare the hollandaise sauce. In a blender, combine the egg yolk, lemon juice, Greek yogurt, cayenne pepper, salt, and pepper. Blend until smooth and creamy. 3. Heat a skillet over low heat. Add the hollandaise sauce and whisk constantly until heated through (do not let it boil). 4. To assemble, place the toasted English muffin on a plate. Top with Canadian bacon, then a poached egg. Drizzle with hollandaise sauce and enjoy! **<u>Nutritional Information (per serving):</u>** Calories: 400, Carbohydrates: 30g, Protein: 25g, Fat: 15g

Servings: 01

**Cooking Time:
10 Minutes**

15. Breakfast Quesadilla

This quick and easy option is perfect for mornings when you're short on time.

Ingredients	Cooking Instructions
<ul><li>1 whole-wheat tortilla</li><li>2 scrambled eggs</li><li>¼ cup shredded cheese (cheddar or Monterey Jack)</li><li>2 tablespoons chopped black beans (optional)</li><li>Salsa and avocado slices (for serving)</li></ul>	<ol><li>Heat a large skillet over medium heat.</li><li>Place the whole-wheat tortilla in the pan.</li><li>Scramble the eggs and spread them over half of the tortilla.</li><li>Sprinkle with cheese and black beans (if using).</li><li>Fold the tortilla in half to create a half-moon shape.</li><li>Cook for 2-3 minutes per side, or until the cheese is melted and the tortilla is golden brown.</li><li>Serve immediately with your favorite toppings like salsa and avocado slices.</li></ol> **Nutritional Information (per serving):** Calories: 350, Carbohydrates: 30g, Protein: 20g, Fat: 15g

CHAPTER 7: Lunchtime Solutions: Quick and Easy Meals for Busy Schedules

Conquering Your Cravings, Not Your Time:

Lunchtime can often be a battle between convenience and healthy choices. This chapter equips you with delicious and satisfying lunch ideas that are perfect for busy schedules, all while keeping your PCOS needs in mind.

We've got options for every taste and dietary preference, including:

- **Quick and Easy Prep:** Perfect for those days when you're short on time in the morning.

- **Leftover Magic:** Transform leftovers into exciting new creations to avoid lunchtime boredom.

- **Salad Sensations:** Explore a variety of flavorful and satisfying salad combinations.

- **Light and Wholesome Soups:** Warm up with nourishing and delicious soups.

Each recipe includes:

- A brief description of the dish

- Preparation and cooking duration

- Number of servings

- Ingredient list

- Step-by-step instructions with easy-to-follow guidance

- Nutritional information, including calories, carbohydrates, protein, and fat

Servings: 01

**Cooking Time:
10 Minutes**

1. Rainbow Veggie Wrap

This vibrant wrap is packed with vitamins, fiber, and protein to keep you feeling full and energized.

Ingredients	Cooking Instructions
1. 1 whole-wheat tortilla 2. ½ cup chopped romaine lettuce 3. ½ cup chopped red bell pepper 4. ½ cup chopped cucumber 5. ¼ cup shredded carrots 6. 2 tablespoons hummus 7. 2 slices turkey breast 8. Salt and pepper to taste	1. Spread the hummus evenly over the whole-wheat tortilla. 2. Layer the romaine lettuce, red bell pepper, cucumber, and carrots on top of the hummus. 3. Add the turkey slices. 4. Season with salt and pepper to taste. 5. Roll the tortilla tightly to create a wrap. 6. Enjoy!

<u>Nutritional Information (per serving):</u>
Calories: 350, Carbohydrates: 30g, Protein: 20g, Fat: 10g

Servings: 01

**Cooking Time:
10 Minutes**

2. Leftover Salmon Scramble

Transform leftover salmon into a protein-packed and flavorful lunch scramble.

Ingredients	Cooking Instructions
1. 2 large eggs 2. 1 tablespoon unsweetened almond milk 3. ¼ cup leftover flaked salmon 4. ¼ cup chopped red onion 5. 1 tablespoon chopped fresh dill 6. Pinch of dried thyme 7. Salt and pepper to taste 8. Non-stick cooking spray	1. In a small bowl, whisk together the eggs and almond milk. Season with a pinch of salt and pepper. 2. Heat a non-stick skillet over medium heat. Coat the pan with cooking spray. 3. Add the chopped onion to the pan and cook until softened, about 2 minutes. 4. Add the flaked salmon to the pan and heat through for another minute. 5. Pour the egg mixture into the pan with the salmon and onions. Let it cook for a minute, then gently scramble the eggs with a spatula until cooked through to your desired consistency. 6. Sprinkle with fresh dill and thyme. Serve immediately. **Nutritional Information (per serving):** Calories:300, Carbohydrates: 5g, Protein: 25g, Fat: 15g

Servings: 02   **Cooking Time:
15 Minutes**

3. Chickpea Salad Lettuce Cups

These flavorful lettuce cups are perfect for a light and satisfying lunch.

Ingredients	Cooking Instructions
1. 1 can (15 oz) chickpeas, rinsed and drained 2. ½ cup chopped cucumber 3. ¼ cup chopped red onion 4. ¼ cup chopped celery 5. 2 tablespoons chopped fresh parsley 6. 2 tablespoons crumbled feta cheese 7. 2 tablespoons olive oil 8. 1 tablespoon lemon juice 9. Salt and pepper to taste 10. 4 large romaine lettuce leaves	1. In a medium bowl, combine the chickpeas, cucumber, red onion, celery, parsley, and feta cheese. 2. In a separate bowl, whisk together the olive oil, lemon juice, salt, and pepper. 3. Pour the dressing over the chickpea mixture and toss to coat. 4. Fill each romaine lettuce leaf with the chickpea salad mixture. 5. Serve immediately. **Nutritional Information (per serving):** Calories: 300, Carbohydrates: 30g, Protein: 15g, Fat: 10g

Servings: 01

**Cooking Time:
10 Minutes**

4. Sunshine Citrus Salad

This vibrant salad is packed with vitamin C and keeps you cool on warm days.

Ingredients	Cooking Instructions
1. 2 cups mixed greens 2. ½ grapefruit, segmented 3. ½ orange, segmented 4. ¼ cup sliced strawberries 5. ¼ cup crumbled feta cheese 6. 2 tablespoons chopped walnuts **For the dressing:** - 2 tablespoons olive oil - 1 tablespoon balsamic vinegar - 1 teaspoon honey - Salt and pepper to taste	1. In a large bowl, combine the mixed greens, grapefruit segments, orange segments, strawberries, feta cheese, and walnuts. 2. In a small bowl, whisk together the olive oil, balsamic vinegar, honey, salt, and pepper for the dressing. 3. Drizzle the dressing over the salad and toss to coat. 4. Serve immediately. **Nutritional Information (per serving):** Calories: 350, Carbohydrates: 35g, Protein: 10g, Fat: 10g

Servings: 01

**Cooking Time:
15 Minutes**

5. Turkey Taco Bowl

This recipe offers a base and endless topping possibility for a flavorful and satisfying lunch bowl.

Ingredients	Cooking Instructions
1. ½ cup cooked brown rice 2. 4 ounces ground turkey, cooked and seasoned with taco spices 3. ½ cup chopped romaine lettuce 4. ¼ cup chopped red bell pepper 5. ¼ cup chopped black beans 6. 2 tablespoons salsa 7. 1 tablespoon crumbled avocado 8. For the optional toppings: - Chopped green onions - Sliced jalapenos - Low-fat Greek yogurt or sour cream - Chopped fresh cilantro	1. In a bowl, combine the cooked brown rice, ground turkey, romaine lettuce, red bell pepper, and black beans. 2. Top with salsa and crumbled avocado. 3. Add your favorite toppings from the optional list, or choose your own! **Nutritional Information (per serving):** Calories: 400, Carbohydrates: 40g, Protein: 30g, Fat: 10g

Servings: 04

Cooking Time: 30 Minutes

6. Lentil Soup with Lemon and Dill

This hearty soup is packed with protein and fiber, making it a perfect choice for a chilly day.

Ingredients	Cooking Instructions
1. 1 tablespoon olive oil 2. 1 onion, chopped 3. 2 cloves garlic, minced 4. 1 teaspoon ground cumin 5. ½ teaspoon dried thyme 6. 1 cup green lentils, rinsed 7. 4 cups vegetable broth 8. 1 can (14.5 oz) diced tomatoes, undrained 9. 1 cup chopped kale 10. ½ cup chopped fresh dill 11. 1 tablespoon lemon juice 12. Salt and pepper to taste	1. Heat olive oil in a large pot over medium heat. Add the onion and cook until softened, about 5 minutes. 2. Add the garlic, cumin, and thyme. Cook for an additional minute, until fragrant. 3. Stir in the lentils and vegetable broth. Bring to a boil, then reduce heat and simmer for 20 minutes, or until the lentils are tender. 4. Add the diced tomatoes with their juices, kale, and dill. Simmer for an additional 5 minutes, or until the kale is wilted. 5. Stir in the lemon juice and season with salt and pepper to taste. 6. Serve hot. **Nutritional Information (per serving):** Calories: 250, Carbohydrates: 30g, Protein: 15g, Fat: 5g

Servings: 01

**Cooking Time:
10 Minutes**

7. Tuna Salad Stuffed Avocados

This recipe takes a classic favorite and transforms it into a healthy and satisfying lunch.

Ingredients	Cooking Instructions
1. 1 ripe avocado, halved and pitted 2. 5 oz canned tuna in water, drained 3. 2 tablespoons chopped celery 4. 1 tablespoon chopped red onion 5. 1 tablespoon light mayonnaise 6. 1 tablespoon lemon juice 7. Salt and pepper to taste	1. In a small bowl, combine the tuna, celery, red onion, mayonnaise, lemon juice, salt, and pepper. 2. Scoop the tuna salad mixture into the avocado halves. 3. Serve immediately. **Nutritional Information (per serving):** Calories: 350, Carbohydrates: 20g, Protein: 25g, Fat: 15g

Servings: 02

**Cooking Time:
15 Minutes**

8. Caprese Chicken Pita Pockets

This recipe is a flavorful and protein-packed option that's perfect for on-the-go lunches.

Ingredients	Cooking Instructions
1. 2 whole-wheat pita breads 2. 4 ounces grilled or baked chicken breast, sliced 3. ½ cup chopped cherry tomatoes 4. ¼ cup crumbled feta cheese 5. ¼ cup chopped fresh basil 6. 2 tablespoons olive oil 7. 1 tablespoon balsamic vinegar 8. Salt and pepper to taste	1. Preheat oven to broil (optional). 2. In a small bowl, whisk together olive oil, balsamic vinegar, salt, and pepper for a simple vinaigrette. 3. Warm the whole-wheat pita pockets in a skillet or the oven on broil for a minute or two (optional). 4. Divide the sliced chicken breast among the warmed pita pockets. 5. Top with cherry tomatoes, feta cheese, and fresh basil. 6. Drizzle with the prepared vinaigrette. 7. Serve immediately. **Nutritional Information (per serving):** Calories: 400, Carbohydrates: 30g, Protein: 30g, Fat: 15g

Servings: 01   **Cooking Time:
15 Minutes**

9. Leftover Veggie Stir-Fry

Transform leftover roasted vegetables into a quick and flavorful stir-fry for lunch.

Ingredients	Cooking Instructions
1. 2 cups leftover roasted vegetables (broccoli, Brussels sprouts, asparagus, etc.) 2. 1 tablespoon olive oil 3. ½ cup chopped tofu, scrambled (or cooked chicken breast for a non-vegetarian option) 4. 1 tablespoon soy sauce 5. 1 teaspoon cornstarch mixed with 1 tablespoon water (to thicken the sauce, optional) 6. Salt and pepper to taste 7. Cooked brown rice (for serving)	1. Heat olive oil in a large skillet over medium heat. Add the leftover roasted vegetables and cook for a few minutes to heat through. 2. Add the tofu (or chicken) and cook until heated through. 3. In a small bowl, whisk together the soy sauce and cornstarch mixture (if using). 4. Pour the sauce over the vegetables and tofu and cook for an additional minute or two, or until the sauce thickens slightly (if using cornstarch mixture). 5. Season with salt and pepper to taste. 6. Serve over cooked brown rice.

<u>Nutritional Information (per serving):</u>
Calories: 350, Carbohydrates: 30g, Protein: 20g, Fat: 10g

Servings: 04

**Cooking Time:
30 Minutes**

10. Creamy Tomato Bisque

This comforting soup is perfect for a cozy lunch on a chilly day.

Ingredients	Cooking Instructions
1. 1 tablespoon olive oil 2. 1 onion, chopped 3. 2 cloves garlic, minced 4. 1 can (14.5 oz) diced tomatoes, undrained 5. 4 cups vegetable broth 6. 1 cup heavy cream (or low-fat Greek yogurt for a lighter option) 7. ½ teaspoon dried basil 8. ¼ teaspoon dried oregano 9. Salt and pepper to taste	1. Heat olive oil in a large pot over medium heat. Add the onion and cook until softened, about 5 minutes. 2. Add the garlic and cook for an additional minute, until fragrant. 3. Stir in the diced tomatoes with their juices and vegetable broth. Bring to a boil, then reduce heat and simmer for 15 minutes. 4. Using an immersion blender or transferring the soup to a blender, puree the soup until smooth. 5. Return the soup to the pot and stir in the heavy cream (or Greek yogurt) and seasonings. 6. Heat through without boiling. 7. Season with salt and pepper to taste. 8. Serve hot. **Nutritional Information (per serving):** Calories: 200, Carbohydrates: 20g, Protein: 10g, Fat: 10g

Servings: 04   **Cooking Time: 20 Minutes**

11. Black Bean Burgers with Chipotle Mayo

These flavorful and protein-packed burgers are a healthy and satisfying lunch option.

Ingredients	Cooking Instructions
1. 1 can (15 oz) black beans, rinsed and drained 2. 1 cup cooked brown rice 3. ½ cup rolled oats 4. ¼ cup chopped red onion 5. 2 tablespoons chopped fresh cilantro 6. 1 tablespoon olive oil 7. 1 teaspoon ground cumin 8. ½ teaspoon chili powder 9. Salt and pepper to taste 10. Hamburger buns (whole-wheat or whole grain recommended) **For the chipotle mayo (optional):** - ½ cup mayonnaise - 1 chipotle pepper in adobo sauce, minced (adjust to preference for spice level) - 1 lime, juiced	1. In a large bowl, mash together the black beans with a fork, leaving some texture. 2. Stir in the cooked brown rice, rolled oats, red onion, cilantro, olive oil, cumin, chili powder, salt, and pepper. 3. Form the mixture into four equal patties. Cover and refrigerate for at least 30 minutes to allow the flavors to meld and the burgers to firm up. 4. Heat a grill pan or skillet over medium heat. Cook the burgers for 5-7 minutes per side, or until cooked through. 5. While the burgers are cooking, prepare the chipotle mayo (optional) by combining mayonnaise, minced chipotle pepper, and lime juice in a small bowl. Adjust the amount of chipotle pepper to your desired spice level. 6. Serve the burgers on hamburger buns with your favorite toppings and chipotle mayo (if using). **Nutritional Information (per serving):** Calories: 400, Carbohydrates: 40g, Protein: 20g, Fat: 15g

Servings: 01

Cooking Time: 15 Minutes

12. Chicken Caesar Salad with a Twist

This recipe uses a lighter Caesar dressing and swaps out croutons for whole-wheat bread cubes for a healthier take on a favorite.

Ingredients	Cooking Instructions
1. 2 cups romaine lettuce, chopped 2. 4 ounces grilled or baked chicken breast, sliced 3. ¼ cup shredded parmesan cheese 4. 2 tablespoons whole-wheat bread cubes, toasted 5. For the light Caesar dressing: - 2 tablespoons olive oil - 1 tablespoon lemon juice - 1 tablespoon grated parmesan cheese - 1 teaspoon Dijon mustard - 1 clove garlic, minced - Pinch of dried oregano - Salt and pepper to taste	1. In a large bowl, combine the romaine lettuce, chicken breast, parmesan cheese, and toasted bread cubes. 2. In a small bowl, whisk together the olive oil, lemon juice, parmesan cheese, Dijon mustard, garlic, oregano, salt, and pepper for the dressing. 3. Drizzle the dressing over the salad and toss to coat. 4. Serve immediately. **Nutritional Information (per serving):** Calories: 400, Carbohydrates: 30g, Protein: 30g, Fat: 15g

Servings: 01   **Cooking Time:
40 Minutes**

13. Quinoa Power Bowl with Roasted Vegetables

This recipe offers a base and endless topping possibility for a protein-packed and flavorful lunch bowl.

Ingredients	Cooking Instructions
1. ½ cup cooked quinoa 2. 1 cup assorted roasted vegetables (broccoli, Brussels sprouts, sweet potato, etc.) 3. 2 tablespoons crumbled feta cheese 4. 1 tablespoon chopped fresh parsley 5. 2 tablespoons balsamic glaze (optional)	1. Preheat oven to 400°F (200°C). Toss your chosen vegetables with a tablespoon of olive oil and roast for 20-25 minutes, or until tender-crisp. 2. While the vegetables are roasting, cook your quinoa according to package instructions. 3. In a bowl, combine the cooked quinoa, roasted vegetables, feta cheese, and fresh parsley. 4. Drizzle with balsamic glaze (if using) and toss to coat. **Nutritional Information (per serving):** Calories: 400, Carbohydrates: 40g, Protein: 20g, Fat: 15g

Servings: 01

**Cooking Time:
10 Minutes**

14. Leftover Turkey Chili

Leftover turkey chili is a perfect way to transform leftovers into a quick and satisfying lunch.

Ingredients	Cooking Instructions
1. 1 cup leftover turkey chili 2. ¼ cup chopped avocado 3. 1 tablespoon chopped fresh cilantro 4. Optional toppings: - Shredded cheese - Sour cream - Chopped red onion	1. In a saucepan, heat the leftover turkey chili over medium heat until warmed through. 2. Pour the chili into a bowl. 3. Top with chopped avocado and fresh cilantro. 4. Add your favorite optional toppings like shredded cheese, sour cream, or chopped red onion for extra flavor and texture. **<u>Nutritional Information (per serving):</u>** Calories will vary depending on the recipe used for the original chili. Refer to the recipe used for the chili for specific nutritional information.

CHAPTER 8: Satisfying Dinners: Nourishing Your Body and Your Taste Buds

Dinnertime Delights

After a busy day, a nourishing and delicious dinner is the perfect way to end the day. This chapter equips you with satisfying and flavorful dinner options designed for busy schedules and PCOS needs.

We've got options for every craving and dietary preference, including:

- **Quick and Easy Creations:** Perfect for those nights when you're short on time.

- **Sheet Pan Suppers:** Minimal cleanup for maximum flavor.

- **Slow Cooker Delights:** Set it and forget it for effortless meals.

- **Comfort Food Classics:** Reimagined with healthy twists to satisfy your cravings.

Each recipe includes:

- A brief description of the dish

- Preparation and cooking duration

- Number of servings

- Ingredient list

- Step-by-step instructions with easy-to-follow guidance

- Nutritional information, including calories, carbohydrates, protein, and fat

So, ditch the takeout menus and grab your apron! It's time to create delicious and <u>satisfying dinners</u> that nourish your body and delight your taste buds!

Servings: 02   **Cooking Time: 20 Minutes**

1. One-Pan Lemon Garlic Salmon with Asparagus

This vibrant sheet pan dinner is packed with protein and healthy fats, all cooked on one pan for easy cleanup.

Ingredients	Cooking Instructions
1. 2 salmon fillets (each about 6 ounces) 2. 1 bunch asparagus, trimmed 3. 1 tablespoon olive oil 4. 1 tablespoon lemon juice 5. 1 teaspoon dried oregano 6. Salt and pepper to taste	1. Preheat oven to 400°F (200°C). 2. In a large bowl, toss the asparagus with olive oil, lemon juice, oregano, salt, and pepper. 3. Arrange the salmon fillets on a baking sheet. Scatter the seasoned asparagus around the salmon. 4. Bake for 15-20 minutes, or until the salmon is cooked through and flakes easily with a fork. 5. Serve immediately. **Nutritional Information (per serving):** Calories: 400, Carbohydrates: 15g, Protein: 30g, Fat: 20g

Servings: 04

Cooking Time: 25 Minutes

2. Sheet Pan Shrimp Fajitas

This colorful sheet pan dinner is bursting with flavor and comes together in under 30 minutes.

Ingredients	Cooking Instructions
1. 1-pound medium shrimp, peeled and deveined 2. 1 tablespoon olive oil 3. 1 teaspoon chili powder 4. ½ teaspoon cumin 5. ¼ teaspoon smoked paprika 6. Salt and pepper to taste 7. 1 bell pepper (any color), sliced 8. 1 red onion, sliced 9. 4 fajita wraps (whole wheat or corn) 10. For the optional toppings: - Guacamole - Salsa - Sour cream - Chopped cilantro - Lime wedges	1. Preheat oven to 400°F (200°C). 2. In a large bowl, toss the shrimp with olive oil, chili powder, cumin, smoked paprika, salt, and pepper. 3. Add the sliced bell pepper and red onion to the bowl and toss to coat with the seasoning. 4. Spread the shrimp and vegetables on a large baking sheet. 5. Bake for 15-20 minutes, or until the shrimp are pink and cooked through. 6. Warm the fajita wraps according to package instructions (optional). 7. Serve the shrimp and vegetables with your favorite toppings like guacamole, salsa, sour cream, chopped cilantro, and lime wedges. **<u>Nutritional Information (per serving):</u>** Calories: 400, Carbohydrates: 30g, Protein: 30g, Fat: 15g (without added toppings)

Servings: 04

**Cooking Time:
4-6 hours on low**

3. Slow Cooker Balsamic Chicken

This slow cooker recipe allows you to come home to a delicious and comforting meal with minimal prep work.

Ingredients	Cooking Instructions
1. 4 boneless, skinless chicken breasts 2. 1 cup low-sodium chicken broth 3. ½ cup balsamic vinegar 4. 2 tablespoons olive oil 5. 1 tablespoon brown sugar 6. 1 teaspoon dried thyme 7. Salt and pepper to taste 8. 1 cup chopped onion (optional) 9. 1 cup baby carrots (optional)	1. In a slow cooker, combine the chicken broth, balsamic vinegar, olive oil, brown sugar, thyme, salt, and pepper. 2. Add the chicken breasts to the slow cooker. 3. Add the chopped onion and baby carrots (if using) to the slow cooker. 4. Cover and cook on low for 4-6 hours, or until the chicken is cooked through and shreds easily with a fork. 5. Serve the chicken with the cooking juices spooned over the top. You can also shred the chicken and serve it over mashed potatoes, rice, or quinoa. **Nutritional Information (per serving):** Calories: 350, Carbohydrates: 5g, Protein: 30g, Fat: 15g

Servings: 04

**Cooking Time:
40 Minutes**

4. One-Pan Lemon Herb Chicken with Roasted Vegetables

This sheet pan dinner is packed with flavor and healthy goodness, all cooked on one pan for easy cleanup.

Ingredients	Cooking Instructions
1. 4 bone-in, skin-on chicken thighs 2. 1 tablespoon olive oil 3. 1 tablespoon lemon juice 4. 1 teaspoon dried thyme 5. ½ teaspoon dried rosemary 6. Salt and pepper to taste 7. 2 cloves garlic, minced (optional) 8. 1 red onion, cut into wedges 9. 1 head of broccoli, cut into florets 10. 1 red bell pepper, sliced	1. Preheat oven to 400°F (200°C). 2. In a small bowl, whisk together olive oil, lemon juice, thyme, rosemary, salt, and pepper. 3. Pat the chicken thighs dry with paper towels. Brush the chicken with the herb mixture. 4. Toss the red onion wedges, broccoli florets, and bell pepper slices with a tablespoon of olive oil and a pinch of salt and pepper. 5. Arrange the chicken thighs in a single layer on a baking sheet. Scatter the vegetables around the chicken. 6. Roast for 35-40 minutes, or until the chicken is cooked through and the vegetables are tender-crisp. 7. (Optional) For crispier chicken skin, broil the chicken for the last few minutes of cooking.

<u>Nutritional Information (per serving):</u>
Calories: 450, Carbohydrates: 30g, Protein: 35g, Fat: 20g

Servings: 04

**Cooking Time:
30 Minutes**

5. Turkey Burgers with Sweet Potato Fries

This recipe uses lean ground turkey and swaps out traditional fries for baked sweet potato fries for a healthier take on a favorite.

Ingredients	Cooking Instructions
1. 1-pound lean ground turkey 2. ½ cup chopped onion 3. ¼ cup chopped fresh parsley 4. 1 tablespoon Worcestershire sauce 5. 1 teaspoon dried thyme 6. Salt and pepper to taste 7. Hamburger buns (whole-wheat or whole grain recommended) 8. For the sweet potato fries: - 2 large sweet potatoes, cut into wedges - 1 tablespoon olive oil - ½ teaspoon paprika - Salt and pepper to taste	1. Preheat oven to 400°F (200°C). 2. In a large bowl, combine the ground turkey, onion, parsley, Worcestershire sauce, thyme, salt, and pepper. Mix gently to combine. 3. Form the mixture into four equal patties. 4. On a baking sheet, toss the sweet potato wedges with olive oil, paprika, salt, and pepper. Spread the wedges in a single layer. 5. Bake the sweet potato fries for 20-25 minutes, or until tender-crisp. Flip the fries halfway through cooking. 6. Heat a grill pan or skillet over medium heat. Cook the turkey burgers for 5-7 minutes per side, or until cooked through. 7. Serve the turkey burgers on hamburger buns with your favorite toppings and the baked sweet potato fries.

<u>Nutritional Information (per serving):</u>
Calories: 450, Carbohydrates: 40g, Protein: 30g, Fat: 20g

Servings: 04   **Cooking Time: 20 Minutes**

6. Creamy Tomato Pasta with Spinach and Goat Cheese

This comforting pasta dish is packed with flavor and protein, making it a perfect vegetarian dinner option.

Ingredients	Cooking Instructions
1. 1-pound whole-wheat penne pasta 2. 1 tablespoon olive oil 3. 1 onion, chopped 4. 2 cloves garlic, minced 5. 1 can (14.5 oz) diced tomatoes, undrained 6. ½ cup vegetable broth 7. 1 cup chopped fresh spinach 8. 4 ounces crumbled goat cheese 9. Salt and pepper to taste 10. Freshly grated Parmesan cheese (optional, for serving)	1. Cook the whole-wheat penne pasta according to package instructions. 2. While the pasta is cooking, heat olive oil in a large skillet over medium heat. Add the onion and cook until softened, about 5 minutes. 3. Add the garlic and cook for an additional minute, until fragrant. 4. Stir in the diced tomatoes with their juices and vegetable broth. Bring to a simmer and cook for 5 minutes. 5. Add the chopped fresh spinach and cook until wilted, about 1 minute. 6. Remove the pan from the heat and stir in the crumbled goat cheese. Season with salt and pepper to taste. 7. Drain the cooked pasta and return it to the pot. Pour the tomato sauce with spinach and goat cheese over the pasta and toss to coat. 8. Serve immediately with freshly grated Parmesan cheese (optional).

Nutritional Information (per serving):

Calories: 400, Carbohydrates: 45g, Protein: 20g, Fat: 15g

Servings: 04   **Cooking Time:
30 Minutes**

7. Salmon with Lemon Dill Sauce and Roasted Asparagus

This dish is perfect for a special occasion or a weeknight meal when you're craving something light and flavorful.

Ingredients	Cooking Instructions
1. 4 salmon fillets (each about 6 ounces) 2. Salt and pepper to taste **For the lemon dill sauce:** - 2 tablespoons olive oil - 2 tablespoons lemon juice - 1 tablespoon chopped fresh dill - 1 teaspoon Dijon mustard - Pinch of dried thyme - Salt and pepper to taste 3. 1 bunch asparagus, trimmed 4. 1 tablespoon olive oil 5. Salt and pepper to taste	1. Preheat oven to 400°F (200°C). 2. Pat the salmon fillets dry with paper towels. Season both sides with salt and pepper. 3. In a small bowl, whisk together the olive oil, lemon juice, dill, Dijon mustard, thyme, salt, and pepper for the lemon dill sauce. 4. On a baking sheet, toss the asparagus with olive oil, salt, and pepper. Spread the asparagus in a single layer. 5. Arrange the salmon fillets on a separate baking sheet. 6. Bake the asparagus for 10-12 minutes, or until tender-crisp. 7. Bake the salmon for 12-15 minutes, or until cooked through and flakes easily with a fork. 8. Brush the salmon with the lemon dill sauce during the last few minutes of baking (optional). 9. Serve the salmon with the roasted asparagus and any remaining lemon dill sauce on the side. **Nutritional Information (per serving):** Calories: 400, Carbohydrates: 15g, Protein: 35g, Fat: 20g

Servings: 04   **Cooking Time: 30 Minutes**

8. One-Pan Honey Garlic Chicken and Brussels Sprouts

This sheet pan dinner is a delightful combination of sweet and savory flavors, all cooked on one pan for easy cleanup.

Ingredients	Cooking Instructions
1. 4 boneless, skinless chicken breasts 2. 1 tablespoon olive oil 3. 1 tablespoon honey 4. 1 tablespoon soy sauce 5. 1 teaspoon Dijon mustard 6. 1 teaspoon dried garlic powder 7. ½ teaspoon ground ginger 8. Salt and pepper to taste 9. 1-pound Brussels sprouts, trimmed and halved	1. Preheat oven to 400°F (200°C). 2. In a small bowl, whisk together olive oil, honey, soy sauce, Dijon mustard, garlic powder, ginger, salt, and pepper. 3. Place the chicken breasts in a single layer on a baking sheet. Brush the chicken with the honey garlic marinade. 4. Toss the Brussels sprouts with a tablespoon of olive oil and a pinch of salt and pepper. Scatter the Brussels sprouts around the chicken on the baking sheet. 5. Bake for 25-30 minutes, or until the chicken is cooked through and the Brussels sprouts are tender-crisp. Baste the chicken and vegetables with the pan juices occasionally during baking. **Nutritional Information (per serving):** Calories: 400, Carbohydrates: 30g, Protein: 30g, Fat: 15g

Servings: 06

**Cooking Time:
8 hours on low or
4 hours on high**

9. Slow Cooker Beef Stew

This slow cooker recipe allows you to come home to a warm and hearty stew with minimal prep work.

Ingredients	Cooking Instructions
1. 1-pound lean stew beef, trimmed and cut into bite-sized pieces 2. 1 tablespoon olive oil 3. 1 onion, chopped 4. 2 carrots, peeled and chopped 5. 2 celery stalks, chopped 6. 4 cloves garlic, minced 7. 1 can (14.5 oz) diced tomatoes, undrained 8. 4 cups beef broth 9. 1 tablespoon Worcestershire sauce 10. 1 tablespoon dried thyme 11. 1 bay leaf 12. Salt and pepper to taste 13. Optional additions: 14. Chopped potatoes 15. Frozen peas	1. Heat olive oil in a large skillet over medium heat. Sear the beef on all sides until browned. 2. Transfer the browned beef to a slow cooker. 3. Add the chopped onion, carrots, celery, garlic, diced tomatoes with their juices, beef broth, Worcestershire sauce, thyme, bay leaf, salt, and pepper to the slow cooker. 4. Stir to combine. 5. Cook on low for 8 hours or on high for 4 hours, or until the beef is tender and the vegetables are cooked through. 6. During the last hour of cooking, you can add optional ingredients like chopped potatoes and frozen peas. 7. Remove the bay leaf before serving. **Nutritional Information (per serving):** Calories: 400, Carbohydrates: 30g, Protein: 30g, Fat: 15g

Servings: 04

**Cooking Time:
20 Minutes**

10. Tex-Mex Turkey Skillet

This one-pan skillet meal is full of bold flavors and healthy ingredients, perfect for a satisfying weeknight dinner.

Ingredients	Cooking Instructions
1. 1-pound lean ground turkey 2. 1 tablespoon olive oil 3. 1 onion, chopped 4. 1 bell pepper (any color), chopped 5. 2 cloves garlic, minced 6. 1 can (15 oz) black beans, rinsed and drained 7. 1 can (4 oz) diced green chiles (mild or hot, depending on your preference) 8. 1 cup chopped tomatoes (fresh or canned) 9. ½ cup low-sodium chicken broth 10. 1 tablespoon chili powder 11. 1 teaspoon cumin 12. ½ teaspoon smoked paprika 13. Salt and pepper to taste **Optional toppings:** - Chopped avocado - Shredded cheese - Sour cream - Chopped fresh cilantro	1. Heat olive oil in a large skillet over medium heat. Add the ground turkey and cook until browned, breaking it up with a spoon as it cooks. 2. Drain any excess grease from the pan. 3. Add the chopped onion, bell pepper, and garlic to the skillet. Cook for 5 minutes, or until the vegetables are softened. 4. Stir in the black beans, diced green chiles, chopped tomatoes, chicken broth, chili powder, cumin, smoked paprika, salt, and pepper. 5. Bring to a simmer and cook for 5-7 minutes, or until the flavors meld. 6. Serve the Tex-Mex turkey skillet with your favorite toppings like chopped avocado, shredded cheese, sour cream, and chopped fresh cilantro. **Nutritional Information (per serving):** Calories: 400, Carbohydrates: 35g, Protein: 30g, Fat: 15g

Servings: 04

**Cooking Time:
25 Minutes**

11. Baked Salmon with Lemon Herb Crust

This recipe is a simple and elegant way to prepare salmon, packed with protein and healthy fats.

Ingredients	Cooking Instructions
1. 4 salmon fillets (each about 6 ounces) 2. 2 tablespoons olive oil 3. 1 tablespoon lemon juice 4. 1 teaspoon dried parsley 5. ½ teaspoon dried dill 6. ½ teaspoon garlic powder 7. Salt and pepper to taste 8. Panko breadcrumbs (optional)	1. Preheat oven to 400°F (200°C). 2. In a small bowl, whisk together olive oil, lemon juice, parsley, dill, garlic powder, salt, and pepper for the herb crust. 3. Place the salmon fillets on a baking sheet lined with parchment paper. 4. Brush the salmon with the lemon herb crust. Alternatively, for a crispier crust, coat the salmon with panko breadcrumbs after brushing with the herb mixture. 5. Bake for 15-20 minutes, or until the salmon is cooked through and flakes easily with a fork. **<u>Nutritional Information (per serving):</u>** Calories: 400, Carbohydrates: 5g, Protein: 35g, Fat: 20g

Servings: 04

**Cooking Time:
30 Minutes**

12. Coconut Curry Shrimp with Vegetables

This flavorful dish is bursting with exotic flavors and uses coconut milk to create a creamy and satisfying curry.

Ingredients	Cooking Instructions
1. 1-pound medium shrimp, peeled and deveined 2. 1 tablespoon olive oil 3. 1 onion, chopped 4. 2 cloves garlic, minced 5. 1 tablespoon curry powder 6. 1 teaspoon ground ginger 7. 1 can (13.5 oz) coconut milk 8. 1 cup vegetable broth 9. 1 bell pepper (any color), chopped 10. 1 cup broccoli florets 11. 1 tablespoon soy sauce 12. Salt and pepper to taste 13. Chopped fresh cilantro (for serving)	1. Heat olive oil in a large skillet over medium heat. Add the shrimp and cook for 2-3 minutes per side, or until pink and cooked through. Remove the shrimp from the pan and set aside. 2. In the same skillet, add the chopped onion and garlic. Cook for 5 minutes, or until the vegetables are softened. 3. Stir in the curry powder and ground ginger. Cook for an additional minute, until fragrant. 4. Pour in the coconut milk and vegetable broth. Bring to a simmer and cook for 5 minutes. 5. Add the chopped bell pepper, broccoli florets, and soy sauce to the simmering curry sauce. Cook for an additional 5-7 minutes, or until the vegetables are tender-crisp. 6. Return the cooked shrimp to the pan and stir to coat with the curry sauce. 7. Season with salt and pepper to taste. 8. Serve the coconut curry shrimp with vegetables over rice or quinoa. Garnish with chopped fresh cilantro for added flavor and color.

Nutritional Information (per serving):
Calories: 450, Carbohydrates: 30g, Protein: 30g, Fat: 20g

Servings: 06

Cooking Time: 40 Minutes

13. Lentil Soup with Sausage

This hearty soup is packed with protein and fiber, making it a perfect cold-weather dinner option.

Ingredients	Cooking Instructions
1. 1 tablespoon olive oil 2. 1 onion, chopped 3. 2 carrots, chopped 4. 2 celery stalks, chopped 5. 2 cloves garlic, minced 6. 1-pound Italian sausage links, casings removed and crumbled 7. 1 cup green lentils, rinsed 8. 8 cups low-sodium chicken broth 9. 1 can (14.5 oz) diced tomatoes, undrained 10. 1 tablespoon dried thyme 11. Salt and pepper to taste 12. Chopped fresh parsley (for serving)	1. Heat olive oil in a large pot or Dutch oven over medium heat. Add the chopped onion, carrots, and celery. Cook for 5 minutes, or until the vegetables are softened. 2. Stir in the minced garlic and cook for an additional minute, until fragrant. 3. Add the crumbled Italian sausage to the pot and cook until browned, breaking it up with a spoon as it cooks. 4. Drain any excess grease from the pot. 5. Rinse the green lentils and add them to the pot along with the chicken broth, diced tomatoes, and dried thyme. 6. Bring to a boil, then reduce heat and simmer for 30 minutes, or until the lentils are tender. 7. Season with salt and pepper to taste. 8. Serve the lentil soup with chopped fresh parsley for garnish. **Nutritional Information (per serving):** Calories: 400, Carbohydrates: 40g, Protein: 25g, Fat: 15g

Servings: 04

**Cooking Time:
20 Minutes**

14. Chicken Stir-Fry with Vegetables

This versatile stir-fry can be customized with your favorite vegetables and protein, making it a great option for busy weeknights.

Ingredients	Cooking Instructions
1. 1-pound boneless, skinless chicken breasts or thighs, thinly sliced 2. 1 tablespoon cornstarch 3. 2 tablespoons soy sauce 4. 1 tablespoon vegetable oil 5. 1 onion, sliced 6. 1 bell pepper (any color), sliced 7. 1 cup broccoli florets 8. ½ cup sugar snap peas 9. ½ cup low-sodium chicken broth 10. 1 tablespoon sesame oil 11. 1 teaspoon sriracha (optional, for added spice) 12. Cooked rice or noodles (for serving)	1. In a bowl, toss the sliced chicken with cornstarch and soy sauce. 2. Heat vegetable oil in a large skillet or wok over high heat. Add the chicken and cook for 3-5 minutes, or until browned and cooked through. Remove the chicken from the pan and set aside. 3. Add the sliced onion and bell pepper to the pan. Cook for 5 minutes, or until the vegetables are softened. 4. Stir in the broccoli florets and sugar snap peas. Cook for an additional 3-4 minutes, or until the vegetables are tender-crisp. 5. Pour in the chicken broth, sesame oil, and sriracha (if using) to the pan. Bring to a simmer and cook for 1 minute. 6. Return the cooked chicken to the pan and toss to coat with the sauce. 7. Serve the chicken stir-fry with vegetables over cooked rice or noodles.

Nutritional Information (per serving):
Calories: 400, Carbohydrates: 30g, Protein: 35g, Fat: 15g

Servings: 04

**Cooking Time:
30 Minutes**

15. Black Bean Burgers with Sweet Potato Fries

These flavorful black bean burgers are packed with protein and fiber, making them a satisfying vegetarian dinner option. Paired with sweet potato fries, they create a complete and delicious meal.

Ingredients	Cooking Instructions
1. For the black bean burgers: - 1 can (15 oz) black beans, rinsed and drained - 1 cup cooked brown rice - ½ cup chopped red onion - ¼ cup chopped fresh cilantro - 2 tablespoons breadcrumbs - 1 tablespoon olive oil - 1 egg (optional, for binding) - 1 teaspoon chili powder - ½ teaspoon cumin - Salt and pepper to taste **2. For the sweet potato fries:** - 2 large sweet potatoes, cut into wedges - 1 tablespoon olive oil - ½ teaspoon paprika - Salt and pepper to taste **3. Optional toppings for the burgers:** - Hamburger buns (whole-wheat or whole grain recommended) - Sliced avocado - Chopped lettuce - Tomato slices - Vegan mayonnaise or your favorite sauce	1. Preheat oven to 400°F (200°C). 2. In a large bowl, mash together the black beans with a fork, leaving some texture. 3. Stir in the cooked brown rice, chopped red onion, chopped fresh cilantro, breadcrumbs, olive oil, egg (if using), chili powder, cumin, salt, and pepper. Mix well to combine. 4. Form the mixture into four equal burger patties. 5. On a baking sheet, toss the sweet potato wedges with olive oil, paprika, salt, and pepper. Spread the wedges in a single layer. 6. Bake the sweet potato fries for 20-25 minutes, or until tender-crisp. Flip the fries halfway through cooking. 7. Heat a grill pan or skillet over medium heat. Cook the black bean burgers for 4-5 minutes per side, or until heated through and browned on the outside. 8. Serve the black bean burgers on hamburger buns with your favorite toppings and the baked sweet potato fries on the side.

Nutritional Information (per serving):
Calories: 400, Carbohydrates: 40g, Protein: 25g, Fat: 15g

CHAPTER 9: Desert Recipes

Sweet Treats You Can Feel Good About: Guilt-Free Desserts

Craving something sweet? Don't worry, you can still indulge without the guilt! This chapter offers a variety of delicious and satisfying dessert options specifically designed for those with PCOS and managing pregnancy cravings. These treats are packed with flavor and use wholesome ingredients that won't spike your blood sugar or leave you feeling sluggish.

We've got options for:

- **Fruity Delights:** Featuring fresh fruit and natural sweetness.

- **Chocolate Fix:** Satisfy your cocoa cravings with healthy alternatives.

- **Creamy Dreams:** Delightful options that are lower in sugar and fat.

- **Frozen Treats:** Cool down with refreshing guilt-free options.

Each recipe includes:

- A brief description of the dessert
- Preparation and cooking duration
- Number of servings
- Ingredient list
- Step-by-step instructions with easy-to-follow guidance
- Nutritional information, including calories, carbohydrates, protein, and fat

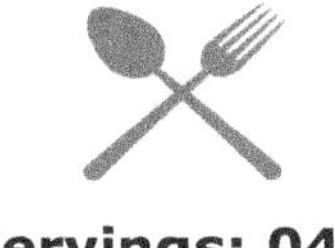

Servings: 04

**Cooking Time:
40 Minutes**

1. Baked Apples with Cinnamon and Walnuts

Warm, spiced apples topped with crunchy walnuts, a simple and satisfying dessert.

Ingredients	Cooking Instructions
1. 4 apples (such as Granny Smith or Honeycrisp) 2. 2 tablespoons lemon juice 3. ¼ cup chopped walnuts 4. 2 tablespoons rolled oats 5. 2 tablespoons brown sugar 6. 1 teaspoon ground cinnamon 7. Pinch of nutmeg (optional) 8. 1 tablespoon melted butter (optional)	1. Preheat oven to 375°F (190°C). 2. Core the apples, leaving the bottom intact. Brush the inside of the apples with lemon juice to prevent browning. 3. In a small bowl, combine the chopped walnuts, rolled oats, brown sugar, cinnamon, and nutmeg (if using). 4. Stuff the apple cores with the oat mixture. 5. Drizzle the melted butter over the apples (optional). 6. Place the apples in a baking dish and bake for 30-40 minutes, or until the apples are tender and the filling is golden brown. **Nutritional Information (per serving):** Calories: 250, Carbohydrates: 40g, Protein: 2g, Fat: 5g

Servings: 04

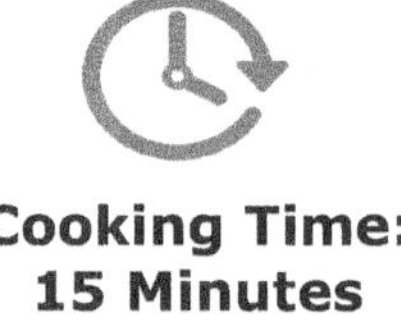

**Cooking Time:
15 Minutes**

2. Dark Chocolate Avocado Mousse

This creamy mousse uses avocado for a healthy fat base and is flavored with rich dark chocolate, perfect for satisfying a chocolate craving.

Ingredients	Cooking Instructions
1. 2 ripe avocados, pitted and peeled 2. ½ cup unsweetened cocoa powder 3. ¼ cup honey or maple syrup 4. 1 teaspoon vanilla extract 5. Pinch of salt 6. ¼ cup milk (dairy or non-dairy) **Optional toppings:** - Fresh berries - Chopped nuts - Coconut whipped cream	1. In a blender or food processor, combine the avocado flesh, cocoa powder, honey, vanilla extract, and salt. Blend until smooth and creamy. 2. Add the milk a little at a time, blending until you reach desired consistency. 3. Divide the mousse between four serving dishes and chill in the refrigerator for at least 30 minutes before serving. 4. Top with your favorite optional toppings like fresh berries, chopped nuts, or coconut whipped cream. **<u>Nutritional Information (per serving):</u>** Calories: 300, Carbohydrates: 30g, Protein: 4g, Fat: 15g

Servings: 04   **Cooking Time:
10 Minutes**

3. Chia Seed Pudding with Berries and Nuts

Prepare this pudding the night before for a quick and healthy grab-and-go breakfast or satisfying dessert.

Ingredients	Cooking Instructions
1. ½ cup chia seeds 2. 1 ½ cups milk (dairy or non-dairy) 3. ¼ cup honey or maple syrup 4. 1 teaspoon vanilla extract 5. Pinch of salt 6. 1 cup fresh or frozen berries 7. ¼ cup chopped nuts	1. In a bowl or jar, whisk together the chia seeds, milk, honey, vanilla extract, and salt. 2. Stir in the berries. 3. Cover and refrigerate for at least 6 hours, or preferably overnight, to allow the chia seeds to absorb the liquid and thicken the pudding. 4. In the morning, stir in the chopped nuts and serve chilled. **Nutritional Information (per serving):** Calories: 300, Carbohydrates: 35g, Protein: 5g, Fat: 10g

 **Servings: 04**

 **Cooking Time: 40 Minutes**

4. Baked Pears with Ginger and Almonds

These baked pears are infused with warming ginger and topped with crunchy almonds for a delightful and satisfying dessert.

Ingredients	Cooking Instructions
1. 4 ripe pears (such as Bosc or Bartlett) 2. 2 tablespoons lemon juice 3. ¼ cup chopped almonds 4. 2 tablespoons rolled oats 5. 2 tablespoons brown sugar 6. 1 teaspoon ground ginger 7. Pinch of nutmeg (optional) 8. 1 tablespoon melted butter (optional)	1. Preheat oven to 375°F (190°C). 2. Core the pears, leaving the bottom intact. Brush the inside of the pears with lemon juice to prevent browning. 3. In a small bowl, combine the chopped almonds, rolled oats, brown sugar, ginger, and nutmeg (if using). 4. Stuff the pear cores with the oat mixture. 5. Drizzle the melted butter over the pears (optional). 6. Place the pears in a baking dish and bake for 30-40 minutes, or until the pears are tender and the filling is golden brown.

Nutritional Information (per serving):
Calories: 250, Carbohydrates: 40g, Protein:2g, Fat: 5g

Servings: 04   **Cooking Time: 2 hours (+ Freezing Time)**

5. Frozen Yogurt Bark with Berries and Granola

This yogurt bark is a healthy and delicious frozen treat perfect for a hot summer day. It's packed with protein and fiber to keep you satisfied.

Ingredients	Cooking Instructions
1. 1 cup plain Greek yogurt 2. ¼ cup honey or maple syrup 3. 1 teaspoon vanilla extract 4. ½ cup fresh or frozen berries 5. ¼ cup granola	1. Line a baking sheet with parchment paper. 2. In a bowl, whisk together the Greek yogurt, honey, and vanilla extract until smooth. 3. Fold in the berries. 4. Pour the yogurt mixture onto the prepared baking sheet, spreading it into an even layer. 5. Sprinkle the granola over the top. 6. Freeze for at least 2 hours, or until solid. 7. Break the frozen yogurt bark into pieces and enjoy!

Nutritional Information (per serving):

Calories: 250, Carbohydrates: 30g, Protein: 10g, Fat: 5g

Servings: 12

**Cooking Time:
10 Minutes**

6. No-Bake Energy Bites with Dates and Nuts

These no-bake energy bites are packed with protein, healthy fats, and natural sweetness, making them a perfect on-the-go snack or satisfying dessert.

Ingredients	Cooking Instructions
1. 1 cup pitted dates 2. ½ cup rolled oats 3. ½ cup chopped nuts (almonds, walnuts, pecans, etc.) 4. ¼ cup unsweetened shredded coconut 5. 2 tablespoons chia seeds 6. 2 tablespoons nut butter (almond butter, peanut butter, etc.) 7. Pinch of salt	1. In a food processor, pulse together the dates until they become a sticky paste. 2. Add the rolled oats, chopped nuts, shredded coconut, chia seeds, nut butter, and salt. 3. Process until well combined and the mixture sticks together. 4. Roll the mixture into tablespoon-sized balls. 5. Store the energy bites in an airtight container in the refrigerator for up to a week.

Nutritional Information (per serving):
Calories: 200, Carbohydrates: 30g, Protein: 5g, Fat: 10g

Servings: 4

**Cooking Time:
10 Minutes**

7. Coconut Chia Pudding with Mango

This creamy pudding is bursting with tropical flavors and healthy fats, perfect for a light and refreshing dessert.

Ingredients	Cooking Instructions
1. ½ cup chia seeds 2. 1 cup coconut milk (full-fat or light) 3. ¼ cup chopped mango (fresh or frozen) 4. 2 tablespoons honey or maple syrup 5. ½ teaspoon vanilla extract 6. Pinch of salt **Optional toppings:** - Fresh mango slices - Shredded coconut	1. In a bowl or jar, whisk together the chia seeds, coconut milk, chopped mango, honey, vanilla extract, and salt. 2. Cover and refrigerate for at least 6 hours, or preferably overnight, to allow the chia seeds to absorb the liquid and thicken the pudding. 3. In the morning, stir the pudding and serve chilled. 4. Top with fresh mango slices and shredded coconut for added flavor and texture (optional). **Nutritional Information (per serving):** Calories: 300 Carbohydrates: 35g, Protein: 4g, Fat: 15g

Servings: 08   **Cooking Time:
40 Minutes**

8.   Sweet Potato Brownies with Pecan Frosting

These brownies are made with sweet potato puree for added moisture and fiber, but still satisfy your chocolate cravings.

Ingredients	Cooking Instructions
1. For the brownies: - 1 cup mashed sweet potato (cooked and cooled) - ¼ cup melted coconut oil - 2 eggs - ½ cup honey or maple syrup - 1 cup unsweetened cocoa powder - ½ cup almond flour - ½ teaspoon baking powder - Pinch of salt 2. For the pecan frosting (optional): - ¼ cup unsalted butter, softened - ¼ cup powdered sweetener (such as Swerve or stevia) - 2 tablespoons chopped pecans - 1 tablespoon milk (dairy or non-dairy)	1. Preheat oven to 350°F (175°C). Line an 8x8 inch baking pan with parchment paper. 2. In a large bowl, whisk together the mashed sweet potato, melted coconut oil, eggs, and honey. 3. In a separate bowl, whisk together the cocoa powder, almond flour, baking powder, and salt. 4. Add the dry ingredients to the wet ingredients and mix until just combined. 5. Pour the batter into the prepared baking pan and spread into an even layer. 6. Bake for 20-25 minutes, or until a toothpick inserted into the center comes out with moist crumbs. 7. While the brownies cool, prepare the frosting (optional). In a bowl, cream together the softened butter and powdered sweetener until light and fluffy. Stir in the chopped pecans and milk until smooth. 8. Spread the frosting over the cooled brownies and enjoy!

<u>Nutritional Information (per serving):</u>
Calories: 250, Carbohydrates: 35g, Protein: 4g, Fat: 10g

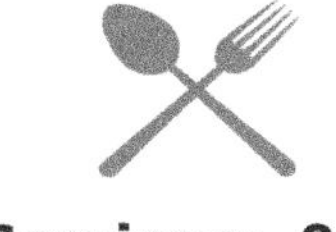

Servings: 04

**Cooking Time:
20 Minutes**

9. Mini Banana Fritters with Honey Yogurt Dip

These bite-sized fritters are made with whole wheat flour and mashed banana for a healthy and satisfying treat.

Ingredients	Cooking Instructions
1. For the fritters: - 1 cup mashed banana (about 2 ripe bananas) - ¼ cup whole wheat flour - 1 tablespoon rolled oats - 1 teaspoon ground cinnamon - Pinch of nutmeg (optional) - ¼ teaspoon baking powder 2. For the honey yogurt dip: - ½ cup plain Greek yogurt - 1 tablespoon honey - 1 teaspoon vanilla extract - Pinch of cinnamon	1. In a large bowl, mash together the bananas. 2. Stir in the whole wheat flour, rolled oats, cinnamon, nutmeg (if using), and baking powder until just combined. 3. Heat a thin layer of oil in a skillet over medium heat. 4. Scoop the batter by tablespoons and flatten slightly into fritter shapes. 5. Cook the fritters for 2-3 minutes per side, or until golden brown and cooked through. 6. While the fritters cook, prepare the dip. In a small bowl, whisk together the Greek yogurt, honey, vanilla extract, and cinnamon. 7. Serve the warm banana fritters with the honey yogurt dip for dipping. **Nutritional Information (per serving):** Calories: 250, Carbohydrates: 40g, Protein: 4g, Fat: 5g

Servings: 8

**Cooking Time:
10 Minutes**

10. Chocolate Chip Cookie Dough Bars

Enjoy this healthier take on a classic treat, with options for both baked and no-bake versions.

Ingredients	Cooking Instructions
1. 1 cup rolled oats 2. ½ cup almond flour 3. ¼ cup unsweetened cocoa powder 4. ¼ cup chopped nuts (such as almonds or walnuts) 5. 2 tablespoons honey or maple syrup 6. ¼ cup nut butter (such as almond butter or peanut butter) 7. Pinch of salt 8. ½ cup chocolate chips (dark chocolate recommended)	1. Preheat oven to 350°F (175°C). Line an 8x8 inch baking pan with parchment paper. 2. In a large bowl, combine the rolled oats, almond flour, cocoa powder, chopped nuts, honey, nut butter, and salt. 3. Stir in the chocolate chips. 4. Press the mixture evenly into the prepared baking pan. 5. Bake for 15-20 minutes, or until the edges are slightly golden brown. 6. Let the bars cool completely in the pan before cutting into squares. **Nutritional Information (per serving):** Calories: 250, Carbohydrates: 30g, Protein: 5g, Fat: 10g

Chapter 10: Snack Recipes

Snacking Smart: Healthy Options to Keep You Going

Eating healthy snacks throughout the day can help you manage your blood sugar levels, curb cravings, and keep you energized during pregnancy. However, with PCOS, it's even more important to choose snacks that are both satisfying and won't trigger blood sugar spikes. This chapter provides a variety of delicious and nutritious snack options that are perfect for busy lifestyles and pregnancy cravings, all while keeping PCOS in check.

We will explore snacks that are:

- **High in Protein and Fiber:** These keep you feeling fuller for longer and help regulate blood sugar.

- **Quick and Easy:** Perfect for those on-the-go moments.

- **Nutrient-Rich:** Packed with essential vitamins and minerals to support your health and your baby's development.

- **Portable:** Easy to take with you wherever you go.

- **Delicious and Satisfying:** Because healthy shouldn't mean bland!

Each recipe includes:

- A brief description of the snack

- Preparation time

- Number of servings

- Ingredient list

- Step-by-step instructions

- Nutritional information, including calories, carbohydrates, protein, and fat

So, ditch the sugary snacks and processed foods, and embrace a world of healthy and delicious options that nourish your body and keep you going throughout your pregnancy!

Servings: 01

**Cooking Time:
10 Minutes**

1. Hard-Boiled Eggs with Edamame

This classic snack is packed with protein and healthy fats, keeping you satisfied and energized.

Ingredients	Cooking Instructions
1. 2 large hard-boiled eggs 2. ½ cup shelled edamame (fresh or frozen) 3. Pinch of sea salt (optional)	1. Boil the eggs for 10 minutes for a medium-hard yolk. Alternatively, purchase pre-cooked hard-boiled eggs. 2. Peel the eggs and cut them in half. 3. If using frozen edamame, cook according to package directions. 4. Enjoy the eggs and edamame together with a sprinkle of sea salt for added flavor (optional). **Nutritional Information (per serving):** Calories: 250, Carbohydrates: 5g, Protein: 15g, Fat: 15g

Servings: 1

**Cooking Time:
5 Minutes**

2. Greek Yogurt with Berries and Chia Seeds

This simple snack is packed with protein, fiber, and antioxidants, making it a perfect choice for a healthy and satisfying treat.

Ingredients	Cooking Instructions
1. ½ cup plain Greek yogurt (2% or higher fat) 2. ¼ cup fresh or frozen berries 3. 1 tablespoon chia seeds 4. Drizzle of honey or maple syrup (optional)	1. In a bowl, combine the Greek yogurt, berries, and chia seeds. 2. Drizzle with honey or maple syrup for additional sweetness (optional). **Nutritional Information (per serving):** Calories: 200, Carbohydrates: 20g, Protein: 10g, Fat: 5g

Servings: 01

**Cooking Time:
2 Minutes**

3. Apple Slices with Almond Butter

This fiber-rich snack is a perfect balance of sweet and savory, and the healthy fats in the almond butter help keep you feeling satisfied.

Ingredients	Cooking Instructions
1. 1 apple, sliced 2. 2 tablespoons almond butter (or other nut butter of choice)	1. Slice the apple into bite-sized pieces. 2. Pair the apple slices with almond butter for dipping. **Nutritional Information (per serving):** Calories: 200, Carbohydrates: 25g, Protein: 3g, Fat: 8g

Servings: 01

**Cooking Time:
2 Minutes**

4. Carrot Sticks with Hummus

This colorful snack provides a satisfying crunch from the carrots and protein from the hummus.

Ingredients	Cooking Instructions
1. 1 cup baby carrots 2. ¼ cup hummus (choose a variety you enjoy)	1. Wash and enjoy the baby carrots with your favorite hummus for dipping. **<u>Nutritional Information (per serving):</u>** Calories: 150, Carbohydrates: 15g, Protein: 4g, Fat: 5g.

Servings: 01

**Cooking Time:
2 Minutes**

5. Cucumber Slices with Cottage Cheese and Everything Bagel Seasoning

This cool and refreshing snack is packed with protein and healthy fats, making it a perfect choice for a light afternoon pick-me-up.

Ingredients	Cooking Instructions
1. 1 cucumber, sliced 2. ½ cup cottage cheese (low-fat or full-fat) 3. Sprinkle of everything bagel seasoning	1. Slice the cucumber into rounds or sticks. 2. Top the cucumber slices with cottage cheese. 3. Sprinkle with everything bagel seasoning for added flavor. **Nutritional Information (per serving):** Calories: 100, Carbohydrates: 5g, Protein: 10g, Fat: 3g

Servings: 01

**Cooking Time:
5 Minutes**

6. Bell Pepper Strips with Guacamole

This vibrant snack offers a satisfying crunch from the bell peppers and healthy fats from the guacamole.

Ingredients	Cooking Instructions
1. 1 bell pepper, sliced into strips (red, yellow, orange, or green) 2. ¼ cup guacamole	1. Slice the bell pepper into colorful strips. 2. Enjoy the bell pepper strips with guacamole for dipping. **Nutritional Information (per serving):** Calories: 150, Carbohydrates: 10g, Protein: 2g, Fat: 8g.

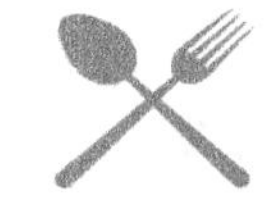 **Servings: 01**

 **Cooking Time: 5 Minutes**

7. Trail Mix with Nuts, Seeds, and Dried Fruit

This customizable snack mix provides a satisfying blend of protein, healthy fats, and fiber.

Ingredients	Cooking Instructions
1. ¼ cup raw almonds or other nuts (cashews, walnuts, pistachios) 2. ¼ cup unsalted pumpkin seeds or other seeds (chia seeds, sunflower seeds) 3. ¼ cup dried fruit (raisins, cranberries, cherries)	1. In a small container, combine the nuts, seeds, and dried fruit. 2. Adjust the proportions of each ingredient to suit your taste preferences. **Nutritional Information (per serving):** Depends on the Ingredients in the Mix.

Servings: 10-12   **Cooking Time:
10 Minutes**

8. Homemade Protein Balls

These protein balls are packed with healthy fats, fiber, and protein to keep you energized throughout the day. They are a great pre-workout snack or afternoon pick-

Ingredients	Cooking Instructions
1. ½ cup rolled oats 2. ¼ cup unsweetened shredded coconut 3. ¼ cup chopped nuts (almonds, walnuts, etc.) 4. 2 tablespoons chia seeds 5. 2 tablespoons nut butter (almond butter, peanut butter, etc.) 6. 2 tablespoons honey or maple syrup 7. ¼ cup dried fruit (chopped dates, raisins, etc.) (optional) 8. Pinch of salt	In a large bowl, combine all ingredients until well mixed. Roll the mixture into tablespoon-sized balls. Place the protein balls on a baking sheet lined with parchment paper. Chill in the refrigerator for at least 30 minutes to allow the balls to firm up. Store the protein balls in an airtight container in the refrigerator for up to a week. **<u>Nutritional Information (per ball):</u>** Calories: 200, Carbohydrates: 25g, Protein: 5g, Fat: 10g.

Servings: 1 - 2

**Cooking Time:
10 Minutes**

9. Roasted Chickpeas with Spices

Roasted chickpeas are a delicious and protein-packed snack that's perfect for satisfying cravings.

Ingredients	Cooking Instructions
1. 1 can (15 oz) chickpeas, rinsed and drained 2. 1 tablespoon olive oil 3. ½ teaspoon cumin 4. ¼ teaspoon paprika 5. Pinch of cayenne pepper (optional) 6. Salt and pepper to taste	1. Preheat oven to 400°F (200°C). 2. In a bowl, toss the chickpeas with olive oil, cumin, paprika, Pinch of cayenne pepper (optional), and salt and pepper to taste. 3. Spread the chickpeas on a baking sheet in a single layer. 4. Roast for 20-25 minutes, or until golden brown and crispy. 5. Let the chickpeas cool slightly before enjoying. **Nutritional Information (per serving):** Calories: 200, Carbohydrates: 20g, Protein: 8g, Fat: 5g.

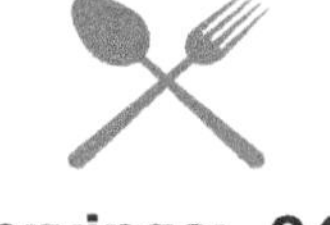

Servings: 04

**Cooking Time:
10 Minutes**

10. Yogurt Bark with Granola and Berries

This yogurt bark is a healthy and refreshing frozen treat perfect for a hot summer day. It's packed with protein and fiber to keep you satisfied.

Ingredients	Cooking Instructions
1. ½ cup plain Greek yogurt 2. ¼ cup honey or maple syrup 3. 1 teaspoon vanilla extract 4. ½ cup fresh or frozen berries 5. ¼ cup granola	1. Line a baking sheet with parchment paper. 2. In a bowl, whisk together the Greek yogurt, honey, and vanilla extract until smooth. 3. Fold in the berries. 4. Pour the yogurt mixture onto the prepared baking sheet, spreading it into an even layer. 5. Sprinkle the granola over the top. 6. Freeze for at least 2 hours, or until solid. 7. Break the frozen yogurt bark into pieces and enjoy! **Nutritional Information (per serving):** Calories: 200, Carbohydrates: 30g, Protein: 10g, Fat: 5g.

CHAPTER 11: Weekly Meal Plans for Different Dietary Needs

Planning healthy and delicious meals throughout the week can be a challenge, especially when managing PCOS and navigating pregnancy cravings. This chapter provides sample weekly meal plans featuring recipes from previous chapters, all tailored to address different dietary needs. Each plan incorporates a variety of the delicious and nutritious options you've discovered, ensuring you stay satisfied and nourished while keeping your PCOS in check.

Important Note: These meal plans are meant as a starting point and can be adjusted based on your individual needs and preferences. Be sure to consult with a healthcare professional or registered dietitian for personalized guidance throughout your pregnancy.

Sample Weekly Meal Plans:

A. Balanced Plate for Overall Wellbeing

This plan emphasizes a balanced approach to nutrition, incorporating a variety of protein sources, healthy fats, and complex carbohydrates.

Monday:

Breakfast: Chia Seed Pudding with Berries and Nuts (Chapter 9, Recipe 3)
Lunch: Sweet Potato Brownies with Pecan Frosting (baked version) (Chapter 9, Recipe 8) and side salad with vinaigrette dressing
Dinner: Baked Pears with Ginger and Almonds (Chapter 9, Recipe 4) with a side of roasted vegetables and quinoa

Tuesday:

Breakfast: Greek Yogurt with Berries and Chia Seeds (Chapter 10, Recipe 2)
Lunch: Apple Slices with Almond Butter (Chapter 10, Recipe 3) and Carrot Sticks with Hummus (Chapter 10, Recipe 4)
Dinner: Hard-Boiled Eggs with Edamame (Chapter 10, Recipe 1) with a whole-wheat toast and a side of steamed broccoli

Wednesday:

Breakfast: No-Bake Energy Bites with Dates and Nuts (Chapter 9, Recipe 6)
Lunch: Trail Mix with Nuts, Seeds, and Dried Fruit (Chapter 10, Recipe 7) with a side of yogurt
Dinner: Roasted Chickpeas with Spices (Chapter 10, Recipe 9) over a bed of mixed greens with a drizzle of olive oil and lemon juice

Thursday:

Breakfast: Smoothie made with spinach, banana, almond milk, and protein powder (not included in recipes)

Lunch: Leftovers from dinner (Baked Pears with Ginger and Almonds) with a side salad

Dinner: Mini Chocolate Chip Cookie Dough Bars (baked version) (Chapter 10, Recipe 10) with a glass of milk

Friday:

Breakfast: Scrambled eggs with chopped vegetables and whole-wheat toast

Lunch: Cucumber Slices with Cottage Cheese and Everything Bagel Seasoning (Chapter 10, Recipe 5) with a side of whole-wheat crackers

Dinner: Bell Pepper Strips with Guacamole (Chapter 10, Recipe 6) with a lean protein source like grilled chicken or fish

Saturday:

Breakfast: Overnight Oats with your favorite toppings (not included in recipes)

Lunch: Enjoy a relaxing brunch! Try avocado toast with a poached egg or a whole-wheat wrap with grilled vegetables and hummus.

Dinner: Coconut Chia Pudding with Mango (Chapter 9, Recipe 7) with a sprinkle of granola for added texture

Sunday:

Breakfast: Pancakes made with whole-wheat flour and topped with fresh fruit (not included in recipes)

Lunch: Leftovers throughout the week

Dinner: Enjoy a family meal! opt for a slow cooker recipe or try a healthy takeout option that aligns with your dietary needs.

B. Vegetarian Delight

This plan caters to those following a vegetarian diet, offering a variety of protein sources from plant-based ingredients.

Monday:

Breakfast: Chia Seed Pudding with Berries and Nuts (Chapter 9, Recipe 3)

Lunch: Sweet Potato Brownies with Pecan Frosting (baked version) (Chapter 9, Recipe 8) with a side of fruit salad

Dinner: Baked Pears with Ginger and Almonds (Chapter 9, Recipe 4) with a lentil soup and a side salad

Tuesday:

Breakfast: Greek Yogurt with Berries and Chia Seeds (Chapter 10, Recipe 2)

Lunch: Veggie Burger on a whole-wheat bun with your favorite toppings and a side salad

Dinner: Hard-Boiled Eggs with Edamame (Chapter 10, Recipe 1) with a veggie stir-fry and brown rice

Wednesday:

Breakfast: No-Bake Energy Bites with Dates and Nuts (Chapter 9, Recipe 6)

Lunch: Trail Mix with Nuts, Seeds, and Dried Fruit (Chapter 10, Recipe 7) with a side of vegetable sticks and hummus

Dinner: Vegetarian Chili with a side of whole-wheat cornbread (not included in recipes)

Thursday:

Breakfast: Smoothie made with spinach, banana, almond milk, and protein powder (not included in recipes)

Lunch: Leftovers from dinner (Baked Pears with Ginger and Almonds) with a side of quinoa salad

Dinner: Mini Chocolate Chip Cookie Dough Bars (baked version) (Chapter 10, Recipe 10) with a glass of plant-based milk

Friday:

Breakfast: Scrambled eggs with chopped vegetables and whole-wheat toast (eggs can be substituted with tofu scramble for a completely vegan option)

Lunch: Bell Pepper Strips with Guacamole (Chapter 10, Recipe 6) stuffed with a black bean and corn mixture in a whole-wheat tortilla

Dinner: Veggie Fajitas with grilled peppers, onions, and your favorite plant-based protein source served on whole-wheat tortillas with all the toppings

Saturday:

Breakfast: Overnight Oats with your favorite toppings and a sprinkle of chia seeds (not included in recipes)

Lunch: Enjoy a relaxing brunch! Try a veggie frittata with your favorite vegetables and cheese (or vegan cheese alternative) or a breakfast burrito with scrambled eggs (or tofu scramble) and vegetables.

Dinner: Coconut Chia Pudding with Mango (Chapter 9, Recipe 7) with a dollop of nut butter and a sprinkle of granola for added texture

Sunday:

Breakfast: Pancakes made with whole-wheat flour and topped with fresh fruit (not included in recipes)

Lunch: Leftovers throughout the week

Dinner: Enjoy a vegetarian restaurant meal or explore a vegetarian version of a global cuisine like Thai curry with tofu or Indian lentil stew (dal) with brown rice.

C. Mindful Portions for Weight Management

This plan focuses on portion control and mindful eating while ensuring you receive adequate nutrients to support your pregnancy.

Monday:

Breakfast: Greek Yogurt with Berries and Chia Seeds (Chapter 10, Recipe 2) with a ½ cup serving of whole-wheat granola

Lunch: Salad with grilled chicken or fish (3 oz serving), a small sweet potato (baked or roasted), and a light vinaigrette dressing

Dinner: Baked Pears with Ginger and Almonds (Chapter 9, Recipe 4) with a controlled portion of quinoa (½ cup) and roasted vegetables (1 cup)

Tuesday:

Breakfast: Scrambled eggs (2 eggs) with chopped vegetables and a slice of whole-wheat toast

Lunch: Apple Slices with Almond Butter (Chapter 10, Recipe 3) and Carrot Sticks with Hummus (Chapter 10, Recipe 4) with a portion control in mind

Dinner: Hard-Boiled Eggs with Edamame (Chapter 10, Recipe 1) with a side of steamed broccoli (1 cup) and a small whole-wheat roll

Wednesday:

Breakfast: No-Bake Energy Bites with Dates and Nuts (Chapter 9, Recipe 6) (limit yourself to 2-3 bites)

Lunch: Trail Mix with Nuts, Seeds, and Dried Fruit (Chapter 10, Recipe 7) with a small portion (¼ cup) and a cup of unsweetened green tea

Dinner: Roasted Chickpeas with Spices (Chapter 10, Recipe 9) over a bed of mixed greens (1 cup) with a drizzle of olive oil and lemon juice

Thursday:

Breakfast: Smoothie made with spinach, banana, almond milk, and protein powder (not included in recipes) with a portion control in mind (limit added sugars from fruits)

Lunch: Leftovers from dinner (Baked Pears with Ginger and Almonds) with a side salad (limit dressing)

Dinner: Mini Chocolate Chip Cookie Dough Bars (baked version) (Chapter 10, Recipe 10) (enjoy 1-2 bars) with a glass of unsweetened almond milk

Friday:

Breakfast: Oatmeal made with whole-wheat oats and topped with a sprinkle of berries (not included in recipes) with a portion control in mind

Lunch: Cucumber Slices with Cottage Cheese and Everything Bagel Seasoning (Chapter 10, Recipe 5) with a small portion of cottage cheese and a handful of whole-wheat crackers

Dinner: Bell Pepper Strips with Guacamole (Chapter 10, Recipe 6) with a lean protein source like grilled chicken or fish (3 oz serving) and a side of steamed green beans (1 cup)

Saturday:

Breakfast: Scrambled eggs (2 eggs) with chopped vegetables and a slice of whole-wheat toast

Lunch: Enjoy a relaxing brunch! Try a one-egg omelet with your favorite vegetables and cheese or a small whole-wheat wrap with grilled chicken or fish (3 oz serving) and a side salad with a light vinaigrette dressing.

Dinner: Coconut Chia Pudding with Mango (Chapter 9, Recipe 7) with a controlled portion (½ cup) and a sprinkle of sliced almonds for added protein

Sunday:

Breakfast: Whole-wheat pancakes (2 pancakes) topped with a small amount of fresh fruit (not included in recipes)

Lunch: Leftovers throughout the week

Dinner: Enjoy a family meal, focusing on lean protein sources and whole grains. Opt for grilled chicken or fish with brown rice and roasted vegetables, or a lentil soup with a whole-wheat bread roll.

These are just samples, and you can adjust portion sizes and meal options based on your individual needs and preferences. Be sure to consult with a healthcare professional or registered dietitian for personalized guidance throughout your pregnancy.

Additional Tips for Meal Planning with PCOS:

- Focus on whole, unprocessed foods.
- Include a variety of protein sources in your diet.
- Choose healthy fats from sources like avocados, nuts, and seeds.
- opt for complex carbohydrates like whole grains and legumes.
- Limit sugary drinks and processed snacks.
- Don't skip meals – aim for small, frequent meals throughout the day to help regulate blood sugar levels.
- Stay hydrated by drinking plenty of water throughout the day.

By following these tips and utilizing the sample meal plans in this chapter, you can create a healthy and delicious approach to eating while managing PCOS and nourishing your body during pregnancy.

CHAPTER 12: Managing Stress for Overall Well-Being

Pregnancy is a joyous time, but it can also be filled with anxieties and uncertainties. This is especially true for women with PCOS, who may face additional concerns about managing their condition alongside the normal challenges of pregnancy. Fortunately, there are many effective strategies you can incorporate into your daily routine to reduce stress and promote overall well-being throughout your pregnancy journey.

Understanding Stress and the Impact on PCOS

Stress is a natural response to challenging situations. It can manifest physically through increased heart rate, muscle tension, and elevated blood pressure. Chronically high stress levels can negatively impact your PCOS symptoms, potentially leading to irregular periods, increased insulin resistance, and worsening mood swings.

Strategies for Stress Management During Pregnancy

Here are some effective strategies to help you manage stress and promote a sense of calm and well-being during pregnancy:

Mind-Body Practices:

- **Mindfulness Meditation:** Taking a few minutes each day to focus on your breath and quiet your mind can significantly reduce stress and anxiety. There are many guided meditation apps and resources available to help you get started.

- **Prenatal Yoga:** Gentle yoga poses specifically designed for pregnancy offer a wonderful way to stretch your body, improve relaxation, and promote better sleep.

- **Deep Breathing Exercises:** Taking slow, deep breaths from your diaphragm is a simple yet powerful technique to activate your body's relaxation response. Practice deep breathing whenever you feel stressed or overwhelmed.

Healthy Lifestyle Habits:

- **Regular Exercise:** Moderate physical activity like brisk walking, swimming, or prenatal fitness classes releases endorphins, natural mood elevators that can combat stress and anxiety. Aim for at least 30 minutes of moderate-intensity exercise most days of the week.

- **Prioritize Sleep:** Getting enough quality sleep is essential for managing stress and overall well-being. Establish a regular sleep schedule and create a relaxing bedtime routine to ensure restful sleep.

- **Healthy Diet:** Eating a balanced diet rich in fruits, vegetables, whole grains, and lean protein provides your body with the necessary nutrients to cope with stress. Limit processed foods, sugary drinks, and excessive caffeine, which can worsen anxiety.

Self-Care Practices:

- **Spend Time in Nature:** Immersing yourself in nature, even for a short walk in a park or sitting by a window with fresh air, can significantly reduce stress and improve mood.

- **Connect with Loved Ones:** Surround yourself with supportive friends and family who understand your journey with PCOS and pregnancy. Talking to loved ones about your concerns can be a great way to de-stress and feel supported.

- **Engage in Activities You Enjoy:** Make time for activities that bring you joy and relaxation, whether it's reading, listening to music, taking a warm bath, or pursuing a hobby.

- **Seek Professional Help:** If you're struggling to manage stress on your own, consider seeking professional help from a therapist or counselor specializing in stress management or pregnancy concerns.

Additional Tips for Managing Stress with PCOS:

- **Stay Organized:** Creating a daily to-do list and prioritizing tasks can help you feel more in control and reduce stress.

- **Learn to Say No:** Don't be afraid to politely decline requests that add unnecessary stress to your already busy schedule.

- **Practice Gratitude:** Focusing on the positive aspects of your life and expressing gratitude can boost your mood and improve your overall well-being.

- **Join a Support Group:** Connecting with other women dealing with PCOS can provide invaluable support, shared experiences, and stress-management strategies.

By incorporating these strategies into your daily routine, you can effectively manage stress, enhance your well-being, and create a more positive and enjoyable pregnancy experience for yourself and your baby.

CHAPTER 14: Building Healthy Habits that Last

Congratulations! You've embraced healthy habits throughout your pregnancy, and now you're preparing for motherhood. This chapter guides you in transitioning those habits into a sustainable lifestyle that benefits you and your growing family.

The Power of Habit Formation

The key to lasting change lies in establishing healthy habits that become ingrained in your daily routine. Our brains thrive on patterns and repetition. By consistently practicing a desired behavior, you create a neural pathway that strengthens over time, making the behavior feel more natural and automatic.

Strategies for Building Sustainable Habits

Here are some key strategies to ensure your healthy habits from pregnancy translate into a long-lasting lifestyle change:

- **Start Small & Celebrate Wins:** Don't overwhelm yourself with drastic changes. Begin with small, achievable goals, like incorporating a daily walk or adding a serving of vegetables to your meals. Celebrate each accomplishment, no matter how minor, to reinforce the positive behavior.

- **Focus on Progress, Not Perfection:** There will be setbacks along the way. Don't get discouraged by occasional slip-ups. View them as learning experiences and recommit to your goals. Remember, progress, not perfection, is the key to long-term success.

- **Make it Enjoyable:** Choose healthy habits you genuinely find pleasurable. Experiment with different recipes, find an exercise routine you love, or explore stress-management techniques that resonate with you. When activities are enjoyable, you're more likely to stick with them.

- **Habit Stacking:** Pair a new habit with an existing one you already perform automatically. For example, listen to a meditation app while walking your dog, or read a book while breastfeeding your baby. This approach leverages existing routines to introduce new behaviors seamlessly.

- **Find an Accountability Partner:** Having a friend, family member, or online support group can provide valuable encouragement and keep you motivated on your journey. Share your goals, celebrate successes, and hold each other accountable for maintaining healthy habits.

- **Focus on the Long-Term Benefits:** Remind yourself of the positive long-term outcomes associated with your healthy choices. This could be improved energy levels, better sleep, weight management, or simply feeling your best. Visualize the future you're creating and let that be your driving force.

Maintaining Healthy Habits with a Newborn

The first few months with a newborn can be a whirlwind. Here are some tips to maintain your healthy habits amidst the chaos:

- **Plan and Prepare:** Plan your meals and snacks in advance to avoid unhealthy choices out of convenience. Prepare healthy snacks and portion out ingredients for easy access.

- **Embrace Short Workouts:** Short bursts of exercise are better than none. opt for brisk walks with the stroller, online fitness classes designed for new moms, or quick yoga routines before the baby wakes up.

- **Delegate and Ask for Help:** Don't be afraid to delegate tasks and ask for help from your partner, family, or friends. This allows you to prioritize self-care and maintain your well-being.

- **Prioritize Sleep Whenever Possible:** Catch sleep whenever your baby naps. This will help you function at your best and have the energy to maintain healthy habits.

- **Find Pockets of Self-Care:** Even small moments of self-care can make a big difference. Take a relaxing bath, steal a few minutes for meditation, or enjoy a cup of tea in a quiet corner. Prioritizing your well-being allows you to better care for your baby.

Building a healthy lifestyle is a journey, not a destination. Embrace the process, celebrate your progress, and be kind to yourself along the way. By incorporating these strategies, you can establish healthy habits that empower you to care for yourself, your baby, and thrive throughout motherhood.

CHAPTER 15: Celebrating Your Journey: Tips for Staying Motivated

Pregnancy with PCOS can be an empowering journey of resilience and self-care. You've embraced healthy habits, navigated challenges, and nurtured your body to create new life. Now, as you approach motherhood, it's crucial to maintain that motivation and celebrate your incredible accomplishments.

The Importance of Staying Motivated

Staying motivated is key to maintaining the healthy habits you established during pregnancy and fostering a positive and joyful experience for yourself and your baby. Here's why motivation matters:

- **Empowers Healthy Choices:** When you feel motivated, you're more likely to make healthy choices regarding diet, exercise, and self-care, ultimately benefiting your well-being and your baby's development.

- **Improves Mood and Reduces Stress:** Motivation fosters a sense of accomplishment and control, contributing to a positive mood and reducing stress levels, both essential for overall well-being.

- **Enhances the Journey of Motherhood:** Staying motivated allows you to approach motherhood with a positive outlook, leading to a more enjoyable experience for both you and your baby.

Strategies for Maintaining Motivation

Here are some effective strategies to stay motivated as you embark on motherhood:

- **Reflect on Your Accomplishments:** Take time to reflect on the incredible journey you've undertaken. Jot down your achievements in a journal, create a visual memory board, or share your triumphs with loved ones. Recognizing your progress fuels motivation to continue.

- **Set Realistic and Achievable Goals:** Break down larger goals into smaller, achievable steps. Celebrate each milestone, no matter how small, to keep yourself motivated and moving forward.

- **Focus on the Positive:** Shift your focus to the positive aspects of healthy habits. Notice how you feel more energized, how your body is adapting, or how your choices are contributing to your baby's well-being. A positive mindset fuels motivation.

- **Find Inspiration:** Surround yourself with positive influences. Seek out inspirational stories of other mothers or connect with online communities focused on healthy living and motherhood.

- **Reward Yourself:** Celebrate your achievements, big or small! Treat yourself to a relaxing massage, a new workout outfit, or a well-deserved night out with your partner. Rewarding progress reinforces positive behaviors.

- **Practice Gratitude:** Cultivate an attitude of gratitude for your body, your health, and the miracle of motherhood. Focusing on what you're grateful for boosts overall well-being and increases motivation.

Building a Support System for Lasting Motivation

A strong support system is crucial for maintaining motivation throughout motherhood. Here's how to build it:

- **Connect with Your Partner:** Discuss your goals and challenges with your partner. Encourage each other and hold one another accountable for maintaining healthy habits.

- **Lean on Family and Friends:** Seek support from loved ones. Ask for help with household chores, childcare, or simply a listening ear. A strong support network provides encouragement and reduces stress.

- **Find a Mommy Tribe:** Connect with other mothers, online or in-person. Sharing experiences, challenges, and successes with others on the same journey fosters a sense of community and motivation.

- **Consider Professional Help:** If you're struggling with motivation or face challenges like postpartum depression, don't hesitate to seek professional help from a therapist or counselor. They can provide valuable guidance and support.

Staying motivated is an ongoing process. There will be days when challenges arise, and that's okay. Be kind to yourself, celebrate your victories, and embrace the incredible journey of motherhood!

CHAPTER 12: Customize Your Meals with Chef-Approved Swaps

Planning healthy and delicious meals throughout pregnancy can be even more exciting when you have options to personalize them! This chapter equips you with chef-approved swap ideas, allowing you to tailor recipes from previous chapters to your specific preferences, dietary needs, or available ingredients.

Embrace Flexibility in the Kitchen

Think of these swaps as a culinary playground! Don't be afraid to experiment and discover flavor combinations that tantalize your taste buds. Remember, the goal is to create delicious and nutritious meals that satisfy your cravings and support your health.

Swapping Protein Sources:

- **Lean Meat Options:** Craving chicken in a recipe that calls for turkey? No problem! Substitute boneless, skinless chicken breasts or thighs for turkey breasts or thighs in most recipes. The same goes for ground turkey; swap it with ground chicken for a similar flavor and texture.

- **Seafood Swaps:** Salmon and shrimp are versatile options. Substitute salmon for cod or halibut in baked fish dishes, or swap shrimp for scallops in stir-fries or kebabs.

- **Plant-Based Protein Power:** Looking for a vegetarian twist? Swap lentils or chickpeas for ground meat in recipes like shepherd's pie or stuffed peppers. Tofu scramble can be a delicious substitute for scrambled eggs in breakfast dishes.

Grains and Carbohydrates:

- **Whole-Wheat Wonders:** Most recipes calling for white rice can be transformed with a swap for brown rice or quinoa, adding fiber and a nutty flavor. Whole-wheat pasta offers a more nutrient-denser alternative to regular pasta.

- **Sweet Potato Power:** Roasting or mashing sweet potatoes creates a delicious and nutritious substitute for white potatoes in dishes like mashed potatoes or potato wedges.

- **Cauliflower Magic:** "Rice" your cauliflower by pulsing it in a food processor for a low-carb, versatile option. Use it in place of rice in burrito bowls, stir-fries, or even sushi!

Fats and Oils:

- **Healthy Oil Swaps:** Substitute olive oil for vegetable oil in most recipes for a heart-healthy alternative. Avocado oil is another great option with a high smoke point for high-heat cooking.

Sweeteners and Spices:

- **Natural Sweeteners:** Swap refined sugar for natural sweeteners like honey, maple syrup, or dates (chopped or pureed) in moderation. These options add a touch of sweetness with additional nutrients.

- **Spice Up Your Life:** Don't be afraid to experiment with different spices and herbs! Add a pinch of cayenne pepper for a kick, or swap dried basil for oregano for a flavor variation. Fresh herbs like parsley, cilantro, or dill add a pop of freshness at the end of cooking.

When swapping ingredients, consider potential adjustments in cooking times or textures. For example, some substitutions might require slightly longer cooking times. Always prioritize your safety and follow proper food handling practices.

Beyond Swaps: Additional Customization Tips

- **Portion Control:** Adjust portion sizes based on your individual needs and hunger levels.

- **Veggie Powerhouse:** Boost the veggie content in most recipes! Add chopped spinach to scrambled eggs, sauteed mushrooms to pasta dishes, or roasted vegetables alongside your main protein.

- **Leftover Magic:** Get creative with leftovers! Leftover roasted vegetables can be added to omelets, chopped chicken can be transformed into a salad topping, or leftover quinoa can be used to create healthy breakfast bowls.

Embrace the Journey of Culinary Exploration

By utilizing these chef-approved swaps and additional tips, you can transform recipes into personalized culinary creations that nourish your body and delight your taste buds throughout your pregnancy journey. Remember, have fun, experiment with flavors, and celebrate the joy of cooking for yourself and your growing family!

Glossary of Terms

This glossary provides definitions for some key terms used throughout this cookbook:

- **Androgens:** Male sex hormones that are also present in women in smaller amounts. Elevated androgen levels are a common characteristic of PCOS and can manifest as symptoms like increased facial or body hair growth, acne, and male pattern baldness.

- **Basal Metabolic Rate (BMR):** The minimum amount of energy your body needs to function at rest. Understanding your BMR can help you determine your daily calorie needs.

- **Blood Sugar:** The amount of glucose (sugar) circulating in your bloodstream. In PCOS, insulin resistance can lead to high blood sugar levels, increasing the risk of type 2 diabetes.

- **Carbohydrates:** Macronutrients that provide your body with energy. Complex carbohydrates, like whole grains, vegetables, and legumes, are preferred over simple carbohydrates like refined sugars and white bread, which can cause blood sugar spikes.

- **Fiber:** A type of carbohydrate that your body cannot digest. It promotes digestive health, regulates blood sugar levels, and aids in feeling full after meals.

- **Follicle Stimulating Hormone (FSH):** A hormone produced by the pituitary gland that stimulates the growth of follicles in the ovaries. In PCOS, FSH levels might be imbalanced.

- **Insulin:** A hormone produced by the pancreas that helps regulate blood sugar levels by signaling cells to absorb glucose from the bloodstream.

- **Insulin Resistance:** A condition where your body's cells become less responsive to insulin, leading to high blood sugar levels. This can contribute to weight gain and other PCOS symptoms.

- **Inflammation:** The body's natural response to injury or infection. Chronic low-grade inflammation is associated with PCOS and may worsen insulin resistance.

- **Leptin:** A hormone produced by fat cells that signals feelings of fullness to the brain. Leptin resistance, common in PCOS, can disrupt feelings of satiety and contribute to weight management challenges.

- **Macronutrients:** Nutrients that your body needs in large amounts for energy: carbohydrates, protein, and fat.

- **Micronutrients:** Nutrients that your body needs in smaller amounts for various functions: vitamins and minerals. Deficiencies in certain micronutrients, like vitamin D, may be more common in women with PCOS.

- **Nutrient Deficiencies:** A lack of essential vitamins or minerals in the body. PCOS can increase the risk of certain nutrient deficiencies due to irregular periods and potential changes in absorption.

- **Ovulation:** The release of a mature egg from the ovary each month. PCOS can disrupt ovulation, leading to irregular periods and fertility challenges.

- **Polycystic Ovary Syndrome (PCOS):** A hormonal condition affecting a woman's reproductive system. Symptoms include irregular periods, excess androgen production, multiple small cysts in the ovaries, and potential complications like insulin resistance and weight management struggles.

- **Stress:** The body's response to physical or emotional demands. Chronically high stress levels can negatively impact PCOS symptoms by disrupting hormone balance and increasing inflammation.

Resources for PCOS Support

Here are some valuable resources to support you on your PCOS journey:

- **National Institutes of Health (NIH):** National Institutes of Health (NIH) website on PCOS https://www.nichd.nih.gov/health/topics/pcos

- **The Polycystic Ovary Syndrome Association (PCOSAA):** A nonprofit organization providing education, advocacy, and support for women with PCOS.

- **Endocrinologist:** A healthcare professional specializing in the endocrine system, which includes hormones and glands like the ovaries. They can diagnose and manage PCOS, as well as any hormonal imbalances.

- **Registered Dietitian (RD):** A qualified nutritionist who can provide personalized dietary guidance to manage PCOS symptoms, improve blood sugar control, and support weight management goals.

- **Support Groups:** Online or in-person support groups connect you with other women managing PCOS, fostering a sense of community and shared experiences. Consider groups like:

- **Verity - The UK PCOS Charity:** https://www.verity-pcos.org.uk/ (UK-based)

- **myPCOSteam:** https://www.mypcosteam.com/resources (online community)

- **Mental Health Professional:** A therapist or counselor can provide valuable support in managing stress, anxiety, or depression that may be associated with PCOS.

Remember, this is not an exhaustive list, and it's crucial to consult with your healthcare professional for personalized guidance and support in managing your PCOS. They can create a treatment plan tailored to your specific needs and health goals.